NO
MAYBE
BABY

NO MAYBE BABY

My Journey through Infertility

MARCY HANSON

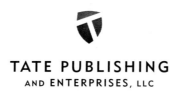

TATE PUBLISHING
AND ENTERPRISES, LLC

Published by Tate Publishing & Enterprises, LLC
127 E. Trade Center Terrace | Mustang, Oklahoma 73064 USA
1.888.361.9473 | www.tatepublishing.com

Tate Publishing is committed to excellence in the publishing industry. The company reflects the philosophy established by the founders, based on Psalm 68:11,
"The Lord gave the word and great was the company of those who published it."

Book design copyright © 2013 by Tate Publishing, LLC. All rights reserved.
Cover design by Rodrigo Adolfo
Interior design by Deborah Toling
Author photo by Mandie Mae

Published in the United States of America

ISBN: 978-1-62510-051-1
1. Family & Relationships / General
2. Family & Relationships / Adoption & Fostering
13.06.10

DEDICATION

To Jon, my husband, my rock. And to Bot Bot, Little Girl, & X-Man, the children of my heart.

CONTENTS

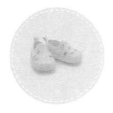

THE BEGINNINGS

Hello, friend! Welcome to my personal journey through infertility and our fight to adopt. The purpose of this book is threefold: I needed a spot to jot down my own thoughts, feelings, and experiences of living with infertility. The second reason is to offer a picture of hope, an understanding ear, and a shoulder to cry on for women and couples who have or are experiencing the battle of infertility, or for those working through the physical implications that come after that final choice to stop trying and come to terms with the fact that there's no more maybe about it—no baby is coming. Finally, it has always been such a strong desire of mine to bring the diagnosis of infertility to a higher level of awareness and shed a little light on the world of adoption. I would love for this book to be a guideline for others who have never dealt with infertility and shed a light of understanding on the multifaceted effects it has on a woman, her husband, and their entire life together. This is my story and how I've come to where I am today. I hope that learning about my journey can help you in some way, if not to only bring light to a topic that is so often considered taboo, but maybe offer you some hope and encouragement that you're not alone in this. We are a sisterhood with no bounds and few who understand.

My journey started about ten years ago. My hubby, Jon, and I were married for about six months when we decided to stop trying to keep from getting pregnant. I'm the youngest of five kids, and never in a million years did I think that we would have any trouble getting pregnant. Granted we were young college students and though not actively "trying" to get pregnant, my constant underlying hope was that we would. To complicate matters, I had started taking the pill about a month before we got married, and as a result when I stopped it, I was incredibly irregular. I would go forty days or so between my periods, so I constantly thought I was pregnant. Let me tell ya, sister, I should own stock in EPT. But every month was the same: no deal. Every month I would think maybe this time, but always the same answer—a big, fat negative sign on the early pregnancy test screen.

We were young, and surely it would come. We just needed to give it time. So time we gave it though I always had this niggling little fear in the back of my mind. After three years my little fear became a downright concern and I started to pay a little more attention to how to get pregnant. It all just seemed so asinine. I mean, really, you have to actively *try* to get pregnant? I didn't have sex until I got married for fear that I *would* get pregnant, and now I had to make a conscious effort to conceive? What in the world was wrong with this picture? I started casually talking to people. At the time I was a hairdresser and I had a client who worked as a registered nurse in an infertility clinic. She became my mainstay of clandestine information. After listening to her heart-wrenching stories about calling couples to tell them that after the thousands of dollars and complete hormone refurbishing they had undergone and still weren't pregnant, I thought it time to see a doctor. So I did. She gave me an exam, ran a series of blood work, and two grand later diagnosed me as perfectly healthy with no reason not to get pregnant should we buckle down and get trying. I started charting temperatures, became addicted to "A Baby Story" on TLC, and planned the nursery in my head.

And what do you know? Still not knocked up. But no one else seemed to be concerned. Our family and friends swore it was stress related. After all, hubby was in graduate school and I had decided to go back to school to be a nurse. Give it time, they all said. But no one had any idea what I was going through. There is an incomprehensible pain that accompanies the desire to get pregnant and the monthly depression that ensues when you don't. Unless you've been there, no one gets it.

That's really the point of this. I want to let you know that I get it. I want to give you my own stories so that you might be able to finally feel like someone can relate. And I want to stop the thought that this is a topic that can't be talked about. This is life. This is real. This is a serious medical condition that affects far more of us than most realize. It isn't shameful, it is painful, and people need to know.

I'm a nurse, and kind of a nerd, so I'll give you some tidbits of facts along the way, but mainly, I just want to chat with you. I hope that in reading this you'll feel like you're sitting down to coffee with an old friend and picking up a conversation that we left off the last time we were together. I don't want to be preachy, and I don't want to be depressing (though as my hubby says, it gets a little heavy at times) so I'll toss in some fun stuff too and hopefully make you smile. I think we're all given our burdens in life, the loads that we carry and weigh us down. For me, my baggage is wrapped in swaddling clothes and strapped to the heart on my sleeve.

Elizabeth Stone once said, "Making the decision to have a child is momentous. It is to decide forever to have your heart go walking around outside your body." But what happens when you make that decision and your heart leaps about waiting for its queue and the feel of the child within you, and the stage call never comes? That is what this story is about. I've cried through it, laughed through it, and prayed through it, and I hope reading it will allow you an opportunity to gain a little understanding or feel not quite so alone. So welcome, friend. Grab a cup of coffee and a piece of chocolate and let's chat. Let me know what you

think, what you'd like to add, and feel free to vent if you need to on the website found at the end of this book. I pray that this is helpful and I look forward to hearing from you!
Take care.

—M

P.S. I've changed names and, in some cases, places throughout this story. I want you to know me and relate to me, but I don't want to put other people in the public eye who may not wish to be so.

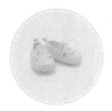

YOU GIVE ME FEVER

Ah baby fever. We've all heard of it, most of us adult women have experienced it, and for some of us, we're in a constant febrile state. I think for the most part we can pinpoint when we first got caught up with getting knocked up. For me, it was right after I got married. My hubby, Jon, and I met in high school. Actually, the first time we met each other, he didn't particularly care for me and I thought he was kind of a jerk. See, he shared a locker with my best friend, and every Tuesday, I would leave pictures or notes for her on the outside of their locker. Why Tuesdays? Well, why not? Jon didn't particularly care for this. In all honesty, he thought it was annoying and told me so, at which point I told him he was just jealous and kind of a jerk (and I'm pretty sure my locker postings might have gotten a little bigger and more frequent after that). After that initial meeting, I didn't really have any contact with him for about a year. He was just that guy who shared a locker with my friend. That all changed our junior year. I was member of the Flathead High Speech and Debate Team (Go, Braves!), and on the ride home from our first meet of the season, I did what any girl stuck on a bus with a bunch of other high schoolers would do: I headed to the back of the bus where the boys were.

There I met Jon again, and this time, I was maybe not so annoying and he was maybe not such a jerk, so much so that we talked the whole five-hour trip back home, finding things that we had in common (and possibly embellishing them a bit too). After that trip, we found ways to meet in the halls and after practice, and before I knew it, I was asking him to the senior ball, our Sadie Hawkins dance. Not long after, on November 14, 1997, he asked me to be his girlfriend, and I said yes. We continued to date through high school and found ourselves on the brink of adulthood and separate paths the summer after our senior year. He was going to be heading off to college and I was getting ready to jump on a jumbo jet and head to Africa on a missions trip. We both knew what was coming; we just didn't know how to broach the topic. Were we going to stay together? Should we call it quits and toss our relationship up to high school love and just move on? Or did we really and truly love each other, even though everyone said we were too young to really know? Well, I'm not one to beat around the bush much, and as summer was coming to an end, I wanted to know where things stood. I knew I loved him and I was willing to tuck it in for the long haul, but I wasn't going to make that commitment if he didn't feel the same way.

So one afternoon, I met him after work and we grabbed a pizza and headed to the park. There, on the swing set of Lion's Club kiddy park, I asked Jon if he was going to marry me some day. Romantic, huh? And maybe a little brazen, but I don't think that's really a big surprise to anyone. He looked at me with his crooked little grin and said "Well, I'd really like to." And that was it. We were in this thing together, come what may. About three weeks later, he took me to Bitterroot Lake, where we loved to canoe and swim, and we watched the sun set behind those beautiful Montana mountains. As it slipped below the ridge, he offered me a small jewelry box with a beautiful promise ring inside. There we made a commitment to each other that regardless of distance and time, I was my beloved's and he was mine.

Just over a year after that, I was home from Africa and enrolled at University of Montana-Western, the same school Jon was attending. We had done a little ring shopping, and I knew when he said he was going to make a trip home to Kalispell to pick up some snow tires, he was really going home to ask my dad for his blessing to marry me.

At that point I was living in a tiny basement apartment with a horrible alcoholic for a landlord. To make matters worse, my landlord lived in the upstairs of the house and one day after a bender, he flew off the deep end and verbally attacked me, ripping up our rental agreement in the process. The next few days were a blur of packing and finding a new place to rent, and I had just sat down to a little TV therapy when Jon called saying he was going to throw some burgers on the grill and I should come over. When I arrived at his house, I was surprised to find the door locked. After knocking loudly and wondering why he had locked the door when he invited me over to dinner, Jon opened the door and all I saw were candles. He had filled every spare inch of his living room with tea lights and tapered candles, setting everything awash in beautiful orange light. He then handed me a card with a picture of a heart on the front, stating that this was his and he would like me to keep it, forever. Through my tears I looked up and found him kneeling in front of me, tears in his own eyes and hands shaking as he said, "I love you with all of my heart. Will you marry me?"

Well, what was a girl to do? I said yes of course! To add to the beauty of the evening, he had made me my favorite dinner, which we enjoyed over candlelight, and then spent the rest of the night calling friends and family to share our exciting news. Though we were over the moon, not everyone was thrilled. After all, we were pretty young, both only nineteen. But it was October and we thought a May wedding would not only be beautiful, it would also bring us both out of our teens to a ripe old age of twenty. And really, it wasn't that far away. When we told my parents that was our plan, I could hear my dad laughing in the background.

"May, huh? That's plan A," he said. "What's plan B?"

The more we thought about it, the wiser my dad became. May really was a long way away, and we were in college so we had a whole month off for Christmas break, why not just get married then? We changed our plan, shook off all the "you're crazy's," and were married young. I was only nineteen and he was twenty—barely. But we'd been together for three years, and when you know, you know. So why wait?

Our ceremony took place among a small group of family and friends in our hometown of Kalispell. I can't tell you how many people told us we'd never make it. We heard it all: you're too young, marriage doesn't last, and it's not real, yadda yadda yadda. But like I said, when you know, you know. We had been married just over a week when I became sick. I was ex-haus-ted. I slept more than I'd slept in my life. I had never been so tired and I had no idea what was wrong with me, so I called my sister. She's pretty much my go-to girl in most situations. A voice of reason, she grounds me pretty well, and she told me I should go pick up a pregnancy test.

This was the first time I had really thought about becoming a mother, and while it scared the heck out of me (I was only nine-teen, remember?), I couldn't help but become excited about the prospect of starting a family. I bought a test—not an easy thing to do for a shy girl (then at least, though now many would beg to differ, my sister the first to make that argument) in a small town where everybody knows your business before you do. But I did it, and with shaking hands and anticipation, I followed the directions, set the timer on my watch, and paced my bedroom for three minutes with my new husband sweating bullets on the couch. Don't get me wrong. Jon would have been ecstatic with the prospect of parenthood, but he's also an itsy-bitsy more rational than I am. The timer goes off, I try and calm myself enough to re-read the directions so I could interpret the results, and there was my sign: No deal. At this point emotions hit me in waves. Part of me was relieved. After all, we were young, poor, in school, and cognitively, I knew it probably wasn't the best timing, but deep down I wanted that pretty little pink + sign more than I had anticipated.

So it began. Baby fever. At this point I was taking the pill, but I also recognized that this wasn't a surefire bet for protection. I knew many people who had babies regardless of their attempts to stay baby-free. To top it off, birth control pills are not my friend. The minute I start taking excess hormones, I start displaying symptoms of pregnancy. The nausea was overwhelming and it got to the point where I could barely cook dinner. When you want to be pregnant, the constant symptoms of being pregnant do nothing but play with your emotions. So at nineteen years old, I caught the fever, and constantly felt pregnant, which made me think I was pregnant. And every month that followed was a big fat slap in the face. Nope. Not this time.

To top it off, my friends were starting to have babies as well. There are such mixed emotions when you want to be pregnant and suddenly everyone around you *is* pregnant. You're excited for them, of course. Really, truly you are. And as excited as you are, your heart is so broken that it's hard to breathe. When you see the pictures of that perfect infant and then hold them in your arms, you can't describe the pain that flows through your veins. This was just the begging. It wasn't a big deal yet, right? I mean, I wanted to get pregnant, but we knew the timing wasn't really perfect. There was no real reason for me to be worried. No one in my family had experienced any difficulty getting pregnant. Quite the contrary. So I tried to let it be and prayed for peace and for patience.

I had no idea the road that this would be, the journey that I was beginning at that tender young age. I had and still have so much to learn and so far to travel, but this was my beginning with baby fever, and this has become so much a part of my life and the woman that I am today.

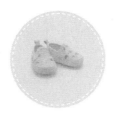

POETRY

I used to write a ton of poetry. Some if it filtered into this journey toward motherhood.

This poem I wrote in the first year we were married as a tribute to the babes I one day hoped to have.

Go to sleep, my little one,
Rest your weary eyes.
Find your slumber in my arms
While I sing a lullaby.
Slip away to dreamland,
On clouds of sugar cream.
Rest away the night time,
Till the dawn light gleams.
The sandman's come to weave his spell,
He's sprinkled fairy dust.
So rest your weary eyes, my joy,
In these arms of love.

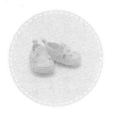

CHEAPER BY THE DOZEN

I recently watched *Cheaper by the Dozen*, the original version. It cracks me up. The little boy who always is trying to sneak a dog home, the teenage girls who are begging to go to the high school dance, the visit from Planned Parenthood, and the chaos that ensues when the children return home from school to find the doctor making a house call, which can only mean one thing: another baby is on the way. Wow, twelve kids. Can you imagine? I remember being in fifth grade and my friend and I were quite sure we were going to have ten children each. It's a nice round number after all. And they would, of course, be born in perfect succession so that each would have a playmate of exactly the same age. But then, as all children do, we grew up and realized that perhaps ten was a bit too round of a number.

I come from a large family. I'm the youngest of five with three brothers and one sister. My husband comes from a small family of two children, he and his sister. Hubby and I decided pretty early that we wanted a pretty large family ourselves. Four little ones sounded like a nicer round number than 10, after all. We had names all picked out even before we officially tied the knot. Our first little boy would be named after my hubby and my father, Jonathan James, and our first little girl would be called Kaliegh Claire. *Kaliegh* is an Irish name meaning "celebration," and what better name than that for our own little celebration?

After that first pregnancy scare right after we were married, we had a good little talk about when would be a good time. Both of us knew that right then wasn't, of course, but still…

I think it became set in stone for me that I was ready for motherhood when Carol, my closest friend in college, had her first baby. I was the first person she told that she was pregnant, and we had so much fun pouring over baby supplies and discussing baby names. After the babe was born, Jon and I gave the new parents a night off and watched the little one while they enjoyed a quiet evening together. I spent the time folding baby clothes, cleaning bottles, and rocking that sweet bundle of new baby joy. I was hooked. To make matters worse, I don't do well on birth control and after six months of marriage, we decided to stop the hormones and quit trying not to get pregnant. At that time I had decided to take a little break from traditional college and attend beauty school. I wanted something more creative in my life and thought that doing hair would be a great way to do that.

I also worked out pretty regularly at the local college's gym and often spent a little quality time on the StairMaster next to a woman who, I swear, was ten months pregnant. Her baby belly was huge! We chatted quite a bit, and it was a shock to me when a few months later, she sat in the chair next to me as I did a client's hair at the beauty school. I asked about the baby and she told me she had a beautiful little girl whom they named Helaina. What a cute name, I had thought to myself and mentioned it to hubby when I got home. He liked it too and we tossed it into the mental name jar.

That following weekend we watched *The Royal Tanenbaums*. Not my favorite movie by a mile, but it has always stuck with me for one reason: at one point in the film, the family boards a stream-liner, and her name was none other than *Helaina*. After that, the coincidences just kept occurring throughout the week. I was working at the time at The Bookstore in Dillon (best bookstore, best boss ever) and had a client come in looking for a book authored by a woman named Helaina. Right after that my boss ordered a book of patron saints, Helaina included. I'm a big believer in watching for signs, and this seemed like a pretty obvious one—we would have a little girl and we would name her Helaina. After all, why so many coincidences over a name I'd never heard of before?

Yes, that was it. Helaina, and we could call her Lainy for short. I had her perfectly imagined in my mind. She would have my husband's chubby baby cheeks and blue-green eyes and my dark curly hair. To make matters worse, Jon and I were both convinced that I was pregnant. I had all the symptoms and the mind plays funny tricks when it comes down to things you desperately want. When the first test came back negative, we waited a couple days and tried again. After the second test yielded the same results, I lost it. Emotionally I was a wreck. I had been so sure that my little Helaina was taking root and we were going to welcome our beautiful girl into the world in just a few months.

My poor husband had no idea what I was going through. He was disappointed, sure, but men don't experience this loss the same way we do. He wasn't emotionally invested like I was, and he shouldn't have been. At this point I was pretty much on my own little battlefield. We weren't officially trying to get pregnant, but I was sure we would be. The poor man, he couldn't do anything right in my eyes, and the truth was he wasn't doing anything wrong. I expected him to comfort me for a loss he didn't know I was grieving, and I was upset when he didn't. It wasn't his fault, and fortunately, he loved me beyond my emotional crisis. Thank God he loves me unconditionally because this was far from the last grieving session.

So here I was—the fever had kicked in, I was off all anti-baby meds, and we had the perfect name with all the signs. Surely, I was going to get pregnant soon and our perfect little family would grow by one. This was further complicated by my own irregularities, and I often thought I was pregnant. Like so many others I've talked to, I would tell myself to wait four more days, and when nothing happened, I'd take a pregnancy test. Every single time, without fail, I would take the test and start the next morning.

I had so many great ideas of how I was going to break the news to my hubby too. I would buy him two cigars, one with a blue ribbon and one with a pink. Or I would buy a onesie and bibs and put them in a little basket with hugs and kisses candy. I also thought about making a little scavenger hunt for him that lead to a Father's Day card, and the list goes on. Once I was so sure I was pregnant, and I had this great idea for a little gift basket for him that I actually took a pregnancy test in the Walmart bathroom (after paying for it of course). But Walmart was an hour from home and I had all the opportunity to buy the supplies for his surprise there, when I didn't back in the small town we were living in. Sounds pretty desperate, huh? Oh sister, believe you me, I was. And I cried the whole way home. We had the names, I had the ideas, we just didn't have the positive pregnancy sign.

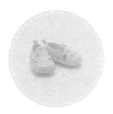

WHAT **NOT** TO SAY

There are so many things that people say to us when we're trying to conceive. Most people think that they are being kind or thoughtful or even encouraging. But here's a little news-flash: most of the time what you think is kind or encouraging is sooooooo not. Here's a few of my favorites:

"Just give it time."

OK, really? Just time, huh? Well, let's see, each day I contemplate exactly where I am in my cycle—if this may be an ovulation day, if I'm even going to ovulate this month, and if I should try to get a little baby making in. In addition, each month I wait twenty-eight days to see if this time I'll get a happy little + sign in the EPT window. And just how many years am I supposed to "just give it time"? Because I seem to remember that when you didn't get pregnant after a month, you about lost your mind.

"You're too stressed. You just need to relax."

Most of the world is stressed. If I could whisk myself away to a sandy beached island and waste away the day eating bonbons and sitting by the ocean, I would. But I happen to be a pretty typical girl who has to work for a living. Silly me, I didn't realize every pregnancy in the history of civilization occurred in times of complete calm and peace.

"You need to lose weight."

French women don't get fat and only skinny chicks get knocked up, huh?

"It's all in God's plan."

Now don't get me wrong. I'm as spiritual as the next girl, and likely a little more, but when all you want is to have a baby, which is a big chunk of our job here on earth, and it doesn't happen, telling me about God's perfect plan makes me a little cranky. I have a pretty strong faith, I understand that he has a master plan, but that doesn't mean it doesn't break my heart. Every. Single. Day.

"But it's OK that you can't get pregnant. God has other children for you."

No, it's not OK. It will never be OK, and I will never be OK. End of story.

"You can always adopt."

You're right. I can, and I did—older children. That doesn't take away the pain. It doesn't change the fact that I will never have a baby shower. That I will never feel my child move within me. That I will never be able to search my child's face and actions for signs of myself, my husband, or other family members. That I will never be the only mommy. That I will not name my own child. That I will never see first steps, hear first words, or decorate a nursery. Granted, had I adopted an infant some of these things would have happened, which leads me to the next point.

"The cost of adoption or IVF is like taking out a car loan."

Actually, it's not. Buying a car means driving off the lot with something tangible. Trying to adopt or doing IVF doesn't necessarily mean that the money you spend results in an infant. Or it may. You may be given an infant, only to wait until the end of a six-month period when the birth mom can go back on her decision and realize that this child is no longer yours, that she wants the baby back. Or wait for years and possibly never receive a placement match. Or put your body through such hormonal hell and your relationship through so much emotional strain that neither of you know if you're going to make it, only to have the pregnancy not take, or miscarry because you are at such high risk. Hormones to get pregnant are not fun, mess with your emotions and cycles, and are pretty much the root of all evil. Oh yeah, that's supposed to be money. Well, they take that too.

"Oh, I know how you feel. My sister/cousin/friend/coworker had the same problem."

Sorry, but you don't know how I feel. Not until you've walked a mile in my shoes and experienced the grieving that I have can you understand. So please, don't try to relate because the truth is, you can't.

"Well, at least you never have to change diapers/do midnight feedings/wonder what they are thinking, etc."

That's your consolation? I would trade anything to be able to rock my baby to sleep in those quiet moments, dreaming about their future and the person they will become. I would feel no greater joy than bonding with my child as I nurse, knowing every inch of their body because I'm the one who bathes them and calms them and changes them.

Things to keep in mind if you happen to be a Fertile Myrtle, or just in general:

I feel like a failure. As a woman, as a wife. Please don't trivialize my pain.

I grieve, every month. Research has shown that women who try to get pregnant and can grieve more for the child they never had than those who have had a child and lost it. Please recognize that this is a real, tangible aspect of my life.

Men want to have a baby; women *need* to have a baby. I don't care about any feminist "we are equal" mumbo jumbo. I want equality as much as the next girl. But the reality is, we as women are hard-wired to be baby makers. When that doesn't happen, there are a whole host of other psychological things that manifest.

Don't exclude me. Don't not invite me to family functions, baby showers, your child's birthday party, or not tell me that you're pregnant because you don't want to hurt my feelings. I can decide if I'm OK enough to attend, but I can't handle it if you exclude me from this part of your life.

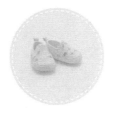

MONKEY IN THE MIDDLE

Do you remember playing the game Monkey in the Middle? There were always at least three people or two teams with one person in the middle. One side would have a ball and toss it to the other side, and the person in the middle was always trying to catch it so they could trade places with someone else. That's kind of what it's like when you're trying to get pregnant. You're the person in the middle while the people on the sides have exactly what they want: the ball. Back and forth it bounces from one person to another, just like pregnancy. Because when you want to be pregnant, I swear everyone around you has a bun in the oven. We had been married two years when this really started sinking in. We hadn't been able to get pregnant, and while a few of our friends had had children, it seemed like all of a sudden, everyone was pregnant. During the time I've tried to conceive, we've had six nieces and nephews, eight cousins (most of whom are like nieces and nephews), and countless friends with babies.

Nothing makes you feel more inept than not being able to get knocked up. I mean, just look at TV. Half of reality television revolves around people getting pregnant and having babies who aren't supposed to (*16 and pregnant*, *Teen Mom*, etc.). And when it seems like every person you know is pregnant, that doesn't help. Last year, my last year of trying, at one point I counted nine friends who had either just given birth or were expecting. Now I know this is the age at which we all try and populate the planet and all, but come on, throw a girl a bone! Like I've said, even though it pains us beyond measure, us Infertile Myrtles really are happy for you—most of the time. Now I know we all have bad days and need to count our blessings and what not, but nothing makes me cranky faster than a pregnant lady complaining about being pregnant. I mean really, for me anyway, it's like a million-aire complaining about having too much money. Let me just dry my tears for you and grab you a box of tissues. We all want what we can't have, right?

At the same time, don't withhold your new mommy news because you're afraid you'll hurt me or make me mad. That's a big reason as to why I'm writing this. People don't talk about infertil-ity because it's uncomfortable and most of us try not to broach the uncomfortable conversations. Unless you're a politician, but that's a whole other story. As a result, so many people are so blind to this issue and how to talk to those of us who live it that all that results is hurt feelings and insecurities. We are, in many situa-tions, very fragile. But we are still your sister, friend, cousin, and we want to share in your joy, through whatever wounds it may open for us.

Here's an example. One of my absolute dearest friends knew that Jon and I had been trying to get pregnant for a while with no success. We had talked about it some, and she knew a lit-tle about infertility through the experiences of one of her family members. She had also had some medical issues of her own and was told that her chances of becoming pregnant were slim to none, so when she became pregnant with her first baby, she was ecstatic. And rightfully so! But here's the hard part: as excited as she was, she didn't want to cause me pain with her news, so she didn't tell me until she was well into her pregnancy. While I totally and completely understand why she withheld, I was so sad at the same time. I had missed out on her initial excitement and the opportunity to share in her joy. So please, don't keep us monkeys in the dark, even though you love us and are trying to spare us further pain. We're pretty good at rebounding. After all, we spend quite a bit of time in the middle.

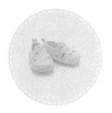

CHANGE OF HEART

After Jon graduated from college and I finished beauty school, we made the biggest move of our young marriage, packed all we owned into an itsy-bitsy U-Haul and moved to Ann Arbor, Michigan. Jon had been accepted to graduate school at the University of Michigan, and while we were excited to start this new chapter in our lives, it was a little terrifying too. After all, we were moving far way from our families and friends to a place where we literally didn't know a soul. But we were young and we were together and that's all that mattered.

We moved into a tiny apartment in married student housing, and before long, I found a job at a salon just a short walk away. The life of a hairstylist in a new area is a difficult one, but I slowly began building my own business and clientele. One of my regulars was a wonderful woman named Beth. She was a registered nurse who worked at a fertility clinic there in Ann Arbor. As nurses, we never seem to be off duty, and I used every appointment with Beth to pick her brain about her job and infertility in general. She was the first person who really opened my eyes to how many people struggle with infertility. But more than that, she is one of the main reasons I decided to go back to school to become a nurse. I loved her confidence and understanding of such a horribly scary issue. I so appreciated her demeanor when she talked about working with her patients and her ability to help others. I wanted that. I enjoyed doing hair, and it was a great way to work while taking classes, but after getting to know Beth, I wanted to be a nurse. And I wanted to work with other people who I so feared were like me.

While I thought I probably fit the niche of the infertile, I still held out hope. One day I asked her what would qualify a person as having fertility issues and her answer cemented my concerns: under twenty-five, active sex life, and not using contraception for one year without a pregnancy. Well, crap. I fit all those things. So I asked a little more about what can be done and how many people really dealt with infertility. What she told me shocked me. She told me at least 1 in 11 women are infertile. That's quite a large number. And the Center for Disease Control says that nearly 10 percent of us can't have babies, and yet what do we hear and know about infertility? Very little. Have you ever tried to look for resources on infertility? I'm kind of a nerd, and I love research, so after talking with Beth I tried to read everything I could get my hands on. In 2003, guess what I found? Very little. Hardly anything online, and libraries were even worse. Still when I go into a library or a book store I check the shelf for recourses and still I am left wanting. Now pregnancy books, that's a different story. The pregnancy bible *What to Expect When You're Expecting* has darn near taken on a cult popularity among mommies-to-be and has expanded through the early years and even to preparations before you get pregnant. And that's not the least of it. Hundreds of books line the shelves on pregnancy and post-partum, how to raise a happy/healthy/strong-willed/genius, and the list goes on and on. But when it comes to fertility, there is little to none.

Remember how I said it's a lonely road? Well, how can it not be when no one even writes resources for us? Why aren't the resources out there? Well, I've got a few ideas on that. For one, it's a difficult topic to discuss; it's kind of the leprosy of motherhood. I swear sometimes when you tell a person you haven't been able to get pregnant, they look at you like it's a catching epidemic and maybe they should step away. Another reason is because it hasn't really been researched all that much. Really only in the last few years has the first batch of longitudinal studies and focus groups on infertility been published. And when it all comes down to it in the doctor's office, it's really just a game of Russian roulette that comes with a big fat price tag. Because once your doc labels your treatments as infertility related (in most cases anyway), you can kiss your insurance contributions to care good-bye.

I have yet to find an insurance company that will assist with the cost of infertility treatments. Here's why: I called and talked with my insurance company at one point to see what all could be covered with this whole baby-making process and was told that once I was coded as having infertility troubles and trying to conceive, the insurance company views those treatments as a "choice" and not necessary for my overall health. As a result, they would no longer continue to cover anything related to those treatments. If I was to become pregnant, then that was fine and they would follow their pregnancy and delivery agreements. If I chose to use birth control or did get pregnant and chose to end the pregnancy, those costs would be covered as well. So the choice to try and get pregnant isn't covered, but the choice to not get pregnant or to end a pregnancy is just fine. Explain to me the logic and hypocrisy behind that.

I've always joked that bartenders and hairstylists are underpaid psychologists, but in this case, I was the patient. I learned from Beth so much about what was potentially happening in my body and what profession was calling my heart. It spurred me on to my own research and inquiries into infertility. It prepared me for what was to come: a long and lonely road, with the opportunity to one day be a voice for others like me.

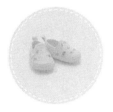

CHARTING

My first visit to the doctors to address our pregnancy concerns was while we were in Michigan. After learning from my client Beth a bit more about infertility, it became pretty apparent that we were likely fitting into that cohort of couples. After doing a little research of my own, Jon and I talked about our potential options and just how far we were willing to go at that point. We decided to start small and look into possible medical issues, hoping of course that there were none.

My friend Jill as was also trying to get pregnant then, and we spent all our time together discussing different ovulation monitoring and tips to getting ourselves into some maternity clothes. My first real, hard-core attempt to monitor and plan a pregnancy, as opposed to just letting it happen, which obviously wasn't working, was to make a little trip to Walgreens. Have you ever walked down that women's isle? I call it that because most men in their right mind wouldn't be caught dead walking those twenty feet surrounded by pink and purple packaging with advertisements for checking your cycles and monitoring your ovulation bombarding them from all sides. My husband avoids it like the plague. It's kind of fun actually to try and trick him into going down the tampon isle when we go grocery shopping. It's even more fun to try and get him to walk down it alone. But I'm kind of a brat like that. Anyway, Walgreens. I had decided that I would start trying to track my ovulation through Basal Body monitoring. It's a pretty simple process really. The principle behind Basil Body monitoring is that your temperature changes minutely through-out your cycle, with the highest spike being at ovulation. All you had to do was keep a thermometer by your bed, and each morn-ing, upon waking, you take your temperature. Here's the stipula-tions: you can't get out of bed and then take it. You can't have a drink of water and then take it. You have to literally roll over with that first fluttering of your lids and pop the thermometer under your tongue. Yeah, easy enough for a morning person, which I am not. I gave it a shot anyway, and as diligently as I could, I kept track of any minute changes in my temperature.

At this time I was working at the salon and, as a result, didn't have health insurance through my job, so our next step was to try and get me some coverage. I searched around and finally found an option that seemed less like a racket than all the other compa-nies and signed myself up. Like I had learned before, it wouldn't cover infertility treatments, but it would help with other medical necessities. Next, I made myself an appointment with a local OB/GYN.

I wanted to get to the bottom of this fertility thing once and for all. After all, Jon and I had made a plan for how we wanted things to roll after we got married. It went something like this: graduate college at twenty-two and get preggo so that our first baby was born when I was twenty-three. After this we would have one child each two years in order to have all four of our ideal little munchkins by the time I was thirty. By now I was twenty-three, nearly twenty-four, and my clock was a tickin'! But you know what they say, if you want to make God laugh, tell him your plans. Well, he must have been rolling up there in heaven because my picture perfect planning certainly wasn't on his agenda. But of course, we didn't know that. So I kept my appointment and went in armed with my concerns and a batch of semi-consistent Basil Body charting.

I liked the doctor I met with well enough, but I wasn't totally impressed. I told her about my concerns with getting pregnant. That we hadn't been using any contraception for quite some time, but I still hadn't been able to get pregnant. She didn't seem to think it was an issue. In fact she acted like I was overreacting and that it wasn't something to be concerned about. She looked at my charting and said that though it didn't seem to show consistent ovulation, everything looked fine. Then she gave me an exam and determined that I was healthy enough to get pregnant, so she'd just order some blood work to rule everything out. The blood work came back fine (and with a big, fat price tag, stupid insurance) and she determined that there was no reason I couldn't get pregnant. Apparently it was all in my head.

I went home not sure what to think. My body seemed to be fine, according to the labs and exam, but I still wasn't ovulating according to my charting. And I certainly wasn't getting pregnant. Still, she thought it wouldn't be a problem, so the rest of our time in Michigan, I spent charting my temperature, doing research, and wondering each month if this would be the month. Soon we were closing that chapter in our lives to make the move to Lewiston, Idaho, and while we were happy to be heading closer to home, I had hoped to be taking a babe home with me.

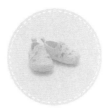

RUBY

I loved the name Ruby. Love it. It conveys the image of a beautiful little girl with rosy cheeks and curly hair, just like I had always pictured our little girl to be. Jon hated it. Well, not hated it, but didn't like it for our baby. He did think it was all right for a dog. So here's what happens when you want a baby and can't have one: you get a puppy. Or in my case, you keep getting puppies until someone give you a child. So when we were offered a beautiful, dark red Golden Retriever by some friends of ours one year at Thanksgiving, I was elated. I was going to have my Ruby, a little something that I could love and nurture, cuddle and snuggle—substituting that new baby smell for puppy breath. By now, Jon and I were in Lewiston and had purchased a little mobile home for our time there. We lived in a little court and had a landlord who had always seemed kind and reasonable. All of our neighbors had dogs, so I didn't think it would be a big deal if we had one as well. After all, we only rented the land from him, and it had a six-foot fence. So when I called to get permission and he shot me down, I was flabbergasted, and my heart was broken. Now I know that many of you may think that I was making a bigger deal out of this than necessary. I can guarantee you that when you want to have a baby and it isn't working for you, your natural desire to mother something, *anything* is far beyond your control. And I lost it.

I remember sitting in my husband's old room at my in-law's house and calling my mom. I told her about the puppy, that it would have been a gift to us, and that my landlord said no. Then I started sobbing. I couldn't understand why if God wouldn't let me have a baby, at least he could let me have a puppy. I know it sounds rather six-year-old and cranky on Christmas, but I was genuinely heartbroken. I didn't think I was asking for that much, and it was just another blow, another loss. I cried the whole six-hour drive home. Then I got mad.

I'm pretty stubborn (ask my husband) and I'm kind of a fighter (ask my brothers). All I had wanted was a puppy for crying out loud, and most of my neighbors had at least one, so why was I any different? I wrote a letter to our landlord. I remember sitting in our computer room, absolutely livid with poison cursing through my veins and fire coming from my ears. You know what they say, hell hath no fury. While I typically have some couth, I'm a bit ashamed to say that it wasn't the nicest letter I've ever written. Granted I wasn't wretched, but I did remind him of all the other animals in the neighborhood, that I was responsible enough to actually ask (I knew for a fact that many of the others around me hadn't received permission), and then I threw in the low blow. I shamelessly filled him in on the fact that we were trying to have a baby, hadn't been able to, and this puppy was my saving grace, which he so heartlessly denied. Oh, I shudder just to think of it. Was he being fair? No, he wasn't. Was I fair? No, not really. In response I received a letter in return stating that we could get a dog so long as it was within a specific size range. (Hurrah for small battles!) So I did what any desperate girl would do: I got a paper and combed the pet ads. And there I found it: free puppies, chow terrier mixes. Jon swore they would be the ugliest thing on earth. I didn't care. As luck would have it, the person with the puppies was just a block from our house and we went over that very night to see them.

The house was disgusting. It was pretty apparent by the trash, dog food, and various other pieces of nastiness that the animals here were not well taken care of. The puppies were kept in the basement of the house all day while the owner worked twelve plus–hour shifts. This was their first time outside. That should give you a nice little picture of their surroundings, and the smell. When he brought them up for us to see (carrying them by the neck), I saw one little girl, and I fell in love. She was a tiny runt of a thing with fuzzy red fur that curled around her ears and dark caramel-colored eyes. And she reeked of neglect. Based on the conditions we wanted to take all of them home, but knew that there was no way we could take more than one, so the little runt came home with us. I put her in the bath first thing when we got back to the house and washed all smell of maltreatment from her soft fur, and we named her Ruby. That night we tried to have her sleep at the end of our bed, snuggled in a towel and blankets, nestled in a laundry basket. But being a puppy and in a new place all alone, she cried and cried. So we (in stupid new puppy parent fashion) brought her up to the bed with us so she could sleep between us.

Ruby nestled her way into our hearts and lives the minute we laid eyes on her. She truly became our first-born, and for the first time during this long and painful journey, she offered a moment of reprieve. We showered her with love and affection, and she returned it tenfold. Where we went, Ruby went, and what we did, Ruby did. I painted the living room and hallway; she tromped around at my feet, covering herself in paint. Every night we went for a walk down on the levy where her floppy little black-tipped ears bounced up and down on her little red head. She lay on the console of my car and sat on my feet so she always knew where if I was going somewhere. It's probably all our fault or maybe a combination of the fact that she and I were both so lost when we found each other, but whatever it was resulted in some serious separation anxiety for Ruby. She couldn't handle it if we left and would cry at the door. One day she got particularly anxious and she ate the arm of our couch. Literally the whole arm was gone, down to the wooden base. I couldn't blame her. When I got home and she was so happy and relieved to see me, my heart just melted. She was my pseudo baby, and I loved her.

I had never understood those people who treated their dog like their child, but at this point in my life, I finally did. It's not that they wanted a dog as a replacement, which could never happen. It's that they wanted something to fill that gaping child-shaped hole in their hearts. For some reason puppy breath seems to do that to an extent. But it doesn't solve the problem. In fact, Ruby wouldn't be our only four-legged addition before we were finally given a child. Three years later, we brought home a bull-headed, big ole beast of a Golden Retriever puppy who we (aptly) named Moose. To us, our dogs are family and a part of who we are and we love them. By the way, it's been eight years since we brought Ruby home, and she still sits on my feet so she knows if I'm going and sleeps between us at night. In a lot of ways, we saved each other.

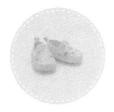

A LITTLE BIT OF THE EAST
FOR THE WESTERNER

It had been a couple of years since my initial doctor's appointment to address our potential infertility concerns, and I still hadn't gotten pregnant. Granted my little Ruby did some good to my soul and eased the pain, I still wanted a baby like nobody's business. I was in the middle of nursing school and though I love nursing care and medicine, I wasn't all that impressed with what I had learned so far about treatments for infertility. I wanted to look a little bit into a more natural route of getting knocked up. After all women have been having babies for thousands of years and someone had to have had the same problems as me and overcome them, right?

I went to our local bookstore and started combing through the nearly nonexistent books relating to infertility and conception. You would think that by 2006, the baby-making industry would have started to address infertility a bit more, but apparently not. I did find one book that I thought was interesting. It was called *The Infertility Cure* and is a guidebook for using ancient Chinese wellness techniques for righting any imbalances in the body to create a suitable environment for pregnancy. In other words, figure out what's up with your yin and yang and get yourself to the maternity ward. I'm in!

I poured over the book, reading different stories of women who had experienced infertility, undergone various medical assistance only to find they were still childless. As a result they turned to Eastern medicine where their hope was renewed and their bodies filled through pregnancy. I learned that Eastern practitioners had a much more holistic view of the body and thus of pregnancy than our clinical Western physicians, to the point that some can even sense a pregnancy through changes in the mother's pulse. In addition, fertility depends on four organ systems: the kidney, spleen, heart, and liver as well as four vital substances: the blood, yang, yin, and qi. These systems and substances can be affected by imbalances within the body, and as a result, a woman experiences the inability to become pregnant.

I was ready to get down and dirty with this new approach, so I took all the questionnaires in the book and resulted in thoroughly confusing myself to the point that I was sure I had it all figured out! I had spleen qi deficiency with liver qi stagnation and dampness. Yep. Made total sense. Now to make it all better. Step 1 was to totally transform my diet. Chubby girls don't get pregnant, apparently. All I had to do with this segment of total body overhaul was to stop eating everything I liked. Hmm, maybe this part wasn't going to work so well. Next I had to go buy me some vitamins. And by some I mean take ownership in the local GNC to keep myself stocked up on things like bee pollen, blue-green algae, and wheatgrass to name a few. Finally I was to find myself an acupuncturist and get poked.

Well, acupuncture for pregnancy certainly wasn't something my new college student insurance covered, so I thought I'd try the other two steps on my own. I tried to revamp my diet and bought some vitamins. But it didn't seem to be working so I decided to look into acupuncturists in our area. I found the perfect one. Our first meeting together I was super impressed. Not only was she an acupuncturist, but she had practiced as a cardiac nurse for thirty-five years before going back to school for chiropractic and acupuncture. It was such a serendipitous event. I don't know if you know anything about nursing school, but it sucks. Period. I was in the midst of clinical and studying and trying to work and get pregnant and all the while questioning if this was really the career path I wanted to take. I knew I wanted to help people, but I also have a huge interest in naturopathic medicine, so could nursing get me there? And here I pulled up in front of this acupuncturist's office and her name on the board is followed by the two little letters I'd been so heavily contemplating: RN. For the first time in longer than I could remember, I felt a little twinkle of hope. But here's the hard thing with hope, just when you get it, it seems to be dashed down again. Like someone rips out your heart, throws it on the ground, and then stomps on it for good measure.

But hope one out and I started seeing my new practitioner regularly. The first appointment was pretty in-depth. She and her assistant asked me a ton of questions about my sleeping habits, pain, and cycles among other things. Then they dropped small amounts of various liquids onto my tongue and asked me to tell them what it tasted like. I have no idea what my responses meant, but there they seemed to tell them quite a bit. After that I began a routine regimen of supplements and vitamins that I purchased from the office. Lord have mercy, at one point I was taking up to thirty-two pills of something a day. But my complexion was wonderful and I was sleeping better than I ever had in my life.

In addition to the supplements, I also started having regular chiropractic work and acupuncture. The chiropractic was sort of expected, my back is all sorts of not right and the acupuncture is what I had originally sought out, though I was nervous for the first session. I quickly learned though that it wasn't anything to be concerned about. The clinic was exceptionally clean and the needles were tiny, so when they were placed I hardly even noticed. After inserting the needles they would hook me up to a small device that would send a small pulsation through wires connecting to the needles. It was only turned up high enough for me to notice and not to cause pain. All in all, it was quite relaxing. They would stick me up like a pincushion, I would pop in my ear buds and clock out of the world for a bit. That is, it was all fine and dandy until one day she decided to fix things up with my ovaries a bit. All of my history with her had revealed that there seemed to be something wrong with this little organ so we were going to address the issue. In order to do so, she inserted a needle into the interior portion of my right ear. I was instantly in tears. Keep in mind I have a pretty high pain tolerance. I'm not generally a wimp and can handle my own, but this was pain like I had never experienced before. Well, that seemed to clarify things a bit. If this Eastern medicine could be trusted, it was pretty apparent that there were some significant issues with my ovaries.

So in addition to the adjustments and acupuncture, they added a few more toppings to my conception Sunday. Soon I was also having regular cleansing foot baths in which I placed my feet in a typical pedicure tub and they placed an ion something-or-other in there with them and supposedly the ion something-or-other would pull all the random toxins in my body out through my feet and cleanse my system. I also started having Erchonia laser treatments to my pelvic area in an effort to fix whatever was going on there. Desperation, remember? Well, after a few months, minimal insurance coverage, more supplements than I could shake a stick at, and a bucket load of money that I couldn't really afford to be spending on all that, I called it quits with this new venture. I was tired of popping so many pills and was losing hope in the obscure additional treatments. Not to mention, I hadn't gotten pregnant. So here I was, back to square one, desperate and getting more and more certain that my only children would be of the four-legged family.

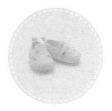

CHILD OF MY HEART

Do you ever watch the TV evangelists? I think my first experiences in this arena were at my grandparent's house. We used to visit my grandpa and step-grandma every summer when we made our annual trip to Oregon. There, we would sit in their little doublewide trailer and my parents would chat, I would play in the orchard, and the TV was always tuned to the Jesus channel. I don't really have any problem with the Jesus channel. I tune in myself on occasion to listen to a little Beth Moore (I can always use a little Moore in my life) and I'm a sucker for any foreign missions trip material. I was a missionary to Africa after all and I hope with all my heart to one day return. But I do tend to think that a good portion of time, they are a little too focus on "me" as opposed to focus on Him. And every now and then, they say something that really makes me angry (I don't believe for a second that the earthquake that rattled Haiti was a direct link to God's anger with the country. I'm pretty sure no one knows who God is displeased with and it certainly isn't my job to judge any one. Just saying.).

At any rate, one day I was taking a little break from my forty hours a week of studying for nursing school and the only thing of moderate interest playing on my whopping five channels was the *700 Club*. I started watching, and when they started praying, I figured why not? Prayer is always a good thing, right? So I closed my eyes, put my hand on my belly, and started praying the same prayer I'd been saying for years. *Please, God, give me a baby.* In the midst of my own concentration, I heard a voice on the TV saying that she had just felt like God was telling her that there were multiple women praying right then to conceive and that "God is going to give you the children of your heart." Well, if that isn't a little coincidental, I don't know what is! But I don't believe in coincidences. I read a book once that said coincidences are God's way of winking at you and I'm pretty okay with that thought. So I watch for signs. After the television host said those words, I instantly started crying and did what I always do in times like that—called my sister.

Name it and claim it, she told me. So I did. My hope was renewed. God had promised me the children of my heart and he in his infinite wonder does not break his promises. Surely, my pregnancy would be quick to follow. I just needed to continue to wait and be patient.

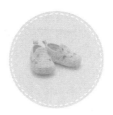

DECEMBER 13, 2006

While everything thus far has been a remembrance of my story, this is an account from my journal:

And Christmas is coming, and once again, we don't have kids. The holidays are so hard, especially when it seems like everyone around me is pregnant or has kids. Kate is due in May; Jessica is do in July (found that out the day after I took a test that was of course negative). And I've found out that a bunch of people from high school have kids. I'm just having a really, really hard time. Especially when I spent this summer getting poked and prodded and downing pills. Then God tells me I'll have the children my heart desires, but that was five months ago, so it's like, okay, I believe you and have faith, but how long is it going to take? Does that mean I'll be like Sarah and Hannah and be old and past my prime before I finally have children? I can't handle that. This last time was horrible—ten full days late, then I spotted for three before starting. You make it that long and think it just may have finally worked. I sobbed for an hour, then Jon cried too. I told him I can't handle this anymore—I'd rather die. And I would. I can't handle this constant pain that only gets worse every day and with each child I see. It's just too much. I can't last.

I honestly don't know if I can face my family and all the kids for Christmas. I don't know if I can handle it. It's too much pain. And I feel like it's never going to get better. And people who haven't dealt with it have no idea what it's like. I feel like I don't have anyone to talk to and it hurts so bad. So bad.

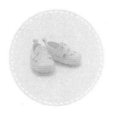

HOLIDAYS

I think that the worst time not to be pregnant or have children is during holidays. Well, except for St. Patty's Day. That's the one holiday you don't want to be pregnant on. But think about it, most of the other holidays are. Mother's Day is the obvious one. I remember sitting in church on Mother's Day Sunday in Michigan, when the church was so beautifully decorated and every mom was on display. Upon entering the foyer, each mom was asked to pick a flower out of one of the many planters and take it into the service with her. After a beautiful message on the beauty of motherhood, each mom walked up the isle to place their flower in a bare wire structure. By the time each flower was placed, the once barren wire structure was filled with petals and the sweet perfume of lilies, roses, and carnations. It was lovely. And I was one of the only women who didn't make that trip down the aisle. Funny how the barren structure became so beautiful. Think of the irony in that one for a minute. Another Mother's Day Sunday I found myself in the pews of our church in Thompson Falls, where one of the young ladies of our church was passing out flowers to each mom in attendance. She tried to hand me a red carnation, and I told her that it was all right, I was not a mom. The sweet girl, she didn't know what to do and obviously didn't want to make me feel bad, so she insisted that I keep the little flower.

Then there's Thanksgiving. Not totally child-centered, but it is a family full event. Not to mention the purpose is to focus on the things you are most thankful for. For me, family has always been on that list. I couldn't wait to teach my children about making a wish on the wish bone or seeing the Thanksgiving crafts they would bring home from school. Not to mention making a little turkey for my little turkeys, who would be running amuck, stealing black olives to put on their fingers, and wrestling for the last piece of pumpkin pie.

While Mother's Day is wretched and Thanksgiving just another reminder, Christmas was the most difficult. After all, one of the major focuses of Christmas is on the children and the whole point of it is based on a miraculous birth. There's no getting away from babies on Christmas. One year, not long after we had been trying, Jon and I were home for the holidays and surrounded by my young nieces and nephews. One night I was sitting on the couch, holding the newest babe in my arms, when my dad leaned over and told Jon with a conspiratorial twinkle in his eye, "She looks good like that, doesn't she?"

Yeah, I did look good like that. I felt good like that. And I wanted that. Do you have any idea how many "baby's first" things there are for Christmas? Baby's first ornament, Christmas outfit, stocking, presents, on and on and on. And unfortunately, asking Santa for a baby for Christmas doesn't seem to work. Trust me, I've tried everything. As Christmas drew closer each year, my anticipation rose. Would this be the year? Would we be able to make the life-changing announcement that we were expecting? Oh, I would hope so! I had so many great ways to break the news to our families. We could frame the first ultrasound and give it to the grandparents-to-be as a gift to unwrap. Or maybe we would buy them a "World's Best Grandparent" mug. Or maybe just break the news at dinner where there would be mass chaos (trust me, my family is huge and Christmas dinner usually has more than twenty people) and lots of tears.

So each Christmas I waited in anticipation. The time would pass when I could hope to provide an ultrasound and continue to travel to the point where I would just pray to be able to make an announcement at dinner. I'm pretty sure that I've taken a pregnancy test every December for the last nine years, just in case. Because Christmas is the story of a miracle, the hope for the hopeless, the birth of a new beginning, each Christmas I hoped for a miracle and I prayed for a birth. Each year one happened in spirit and in heart. The dawning of the new year brought a new focus and wish: maybe this would be the year.

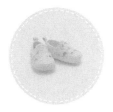

NEW SPECIALIST

My fourth semester of nursing school brought multiple changes. For one, Jon was offered a job working for Montana Fish Wildlife and Parks, which meant that he could no longer live in Idaho, but I still had a year and a half of school to complete. So we made some pretty major changes. We put our little trailer up for sale and he moved to Thompson Falls to start his new job. At this point I was becoming resigned to the fact that the only way we were going to get those children of my heart was through adoption. I had looked into adoption agencies and options a bit in the past and even requested some information, but I felt I was really at the point where it was our own viable option, so I broached the topic with Jon and we decided to request some information from Bethany adoption resources. My whole life I had felt that though I wanted to have biological children, I was meant to adopt as well.

I was so excited the day we got the packet in the mail. I opened the manila envelope to find glossy pages of children in foreign countries who were waiting for someone to take them home. I also learned about home studies and social workers and adoption prices based on country specification. It was so overwhelming, but so exciting at the same time and I couldn't wait to share it with Jon.

That evening we were headed the two hours home to Kalispell to visit our family. As the car is typically when we have our major conversations (I'm serious. We discussed whether or not we were in love when we were seventeen and driving home from a weekend visiting family in Troy), I bombarded him with pamphlets and pictures and started discussing the advantages of adopting from Guatemala as opposed to China, and all of the things we had to do to become eligible to adopt. I may have overwhelmed him. I've been known to get a little intense at times. I get it from a couple of my brothers.

"So what do you think about Guatemala?" I asked. "The children are in foster homes instead of orphanages like in most of the other countries. Also, the price isn't as much as many of the European countries either."

"I don't know," Jon replied. "What do you think?"

"Well, I think there are lots of different options we can take and ways to get monetary assistance that we can look into also. Then we have to also think about home studies and everything that entails as well. Most of these places want a good portion of the money up front, and I don't think we have it."

Silence. "So what do you think?" I asked again.

"I don't know. I'm not sure if we should do this yet."

"What aren't you sure about?" I asked, starting to panic. I thought we were on the same page, after all.

"Well, I'm just not sure if we've tried everything for us to get pregnant."

"What else do you want to try?"

"Maybe we should see a specialist. I think our insurance now will cover it, and it's worth a try," Jon said.

"Okay," I said, dumbfounded.

Granted to this point our insurance hadn't covered anything and all my treatments had been out of pocket, but it still seemed out of reach. "If that's what you want to do, I'll look into specialists and insurance coverage."

So I did. I found a specialist APRN in Kalispell that our insurance would cover and seemed to have a pretty good run of things when it came to dealing with infertility. The problem was that not only was she two hours from our new home in Thompson Falls, but I was still in school in Idaho for the remainder of the semester. That meant that with each appointment I booked, I drove at least two and sometimes six hours to make it. Based on how much I've had to commute in my life, cars should run and hide when I walk on the lot.

My first visit with the new specialist was good. I really liked the clinic. It was peaceful and clean and the office staff was incredibly friendly. The nurse practitioner seemed to be pretty great as well. She did a comprehensive exam, ordered some blood work, and had me schedule an appointment for Jon and me to return for a consultation with their staff and an ultrasound for me. I was excited for the ultrasound, hoping that it would tell us a bit more about what was going on, and pictured my bare belly cooling with the application of the thick blue gel, and maybe beyond miracles, there would magically be a heartbeat! Oh, the thing of dreams!

That is not what happened. There was no abdominal ultrasound. She wanted to do an internal scan instead. Awesome. But she was able to offer some answers. It looked like while my uterus appeared to be of normal size and look okay, my ovaries had multiple cysts. For the first time, I had a diagnosis: Polycystic Ovarian Syndrome (PCOS). She told me not to worry. There are plenty of people with PCOS who have pregnancy success stories and I didn't appear to be on the drastic end of the spectrum: no facial hair, but I did have some issues with my complexion, and while I'd never been really big, I'd always been heavier than I had wanted regardless of exercise. Our next stop was to talk with one of their assistants about PCOS and what it can entail as far as treatment. We would be coming back to the office to do a little more evaluation, and then she would be prescribing my first dose of fertility medications: Clomid. In addition, Jon would need to provide a sperm sample to make sure that all was well in that department.

A couple of weeks later, I returned and she prepped me for another exam, this time in which she utilized the internal ultrasound to monitor a saline flush, testing for patency of my fallopian tubes. Talk about uncomfortable. And to top it off, the tube went in a bit too far and bruised the top of my uterus, causing extreme cramping and pain. Awesome. But my tubes looked good, so it seemed like the Clomid should work just fine at stimulating my ovaries to ovulate and my fallopian tubes should be just fine to carry on the next step of fertilization. With a new prescription in my hand, encouragement that we would be parents within the next six months, and a few warnings (may cause hot flashes and increases your potential for twins), I left the office excited and hopeful. Even the pharmacist at Shopko had my back, telling me he'd seen Clomid be successful for many women in his career. Now I just waited for days five through nine of my cycle to take my first 25mg dose.

On day 10, I was to start using ovulation prediction kits, and on day 12, I was to go in and have a blood draw to see where my hormone levels were and if the Clomid was doing its job. The labs came back and so far, so good! Now I just had to wait and see if it worked or not. So I did, and I waited, and no deal. But she had given me a prescription for three months so I steeled myself for two more cycles, after which I was to return for another exam. Here's the great thing about Clomid: while it stimulates ovulation, it also increases your chance for ovarian cysts. I was damned if I did, and damned if I didn't. But I wanted a baby, so I was willing to take this step.

After the third month I returned for my follow-up exam. I waited in the waiting room for two hours. I know it's not necessarily their fault and likely just some poor scheduling, but making a hormonal lady trying to get pregnant who just drove two hours to be there wait isn't the best idea. But I waited and my ultrasound showed that I still had cysts and still didn't have a magical little heartbeat. We tried for another three months and she reminded me to tell Jon to bring in a sample. The next three months yielded the same results and though I was scheduled for another exam, I didn't go. Jon had never taken in a sample and as far as I was concerned, he was the one who wanted to take this next step. I had been poked and prodded enough.

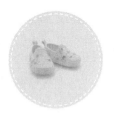

BE STILL

I'll be the first to say that when it gets right down to it, this whole process has made me sad, angry, disheartened, and downright pissed off. And not just at life in general, but at God too. I mean, I've worked with a lot of people in my life, and a lot of people that can't or won't provide for their kids. I've instituted programs to battle childhood hunger and improve nutrition and life choices. I've lived a life I hope to be proud of. I work hard, I have good morals, I try and follow the wisdom of the Word and create a stronger spiritual relationship. And darn it, I deserve to be pregnant! Look at all the women out there who have babies and drink, smoke, or do drugs during their pregnancy. Look at all the parents who cause irreparable mental, physical, or emotional harm to a child due to their own selfishness. Check out your local high school and see how many girls are pregnant or home with a baby when they should be out at the homecoming game. I wasn't that girl, that mom-to-be, that parent, so why has this fundamental thing been withheld from me?

Well, therein lays the little golden nugget. Look back over that previous paragraph and see how many times I say *I* or *me*. A lot. Here's the reality: infertility didn't happen to me because of something Jon or I did or didn't do. It doesn't discriminate between the wealthy, middle class, or the poor. It doesn't differentiate between my good works or those of the girl down the street.

So why did it happen to me, or to you for that matter? The truth is that I honestly don't know. I don't know why God allows bad things to happen to good people, but I imagine it lays somewhere along the lines of the fact that we live in a dangerous world. I also know that there came a time in my life when I had to just suck it up.

I watched the television show *19 and Counting*. If you haven't seen it, I'm sure that you've heard of it: the Duggar family with their brood of children that always seems to be growing. There have been times in my life when I've been insanely jealous of the mom, Michelle. Not because I want my children to number the double digits. Lord no, I like my sanity and I know myself better than that. But because it's another case of the just-not-fairs. It's not fair that I can't even get pregnant, will never feel the movement of a child within me, and she's been pregnant twenty-one times. While I don't believe her extensive ability to carry children has to do with her "goodness" or the strength of her relationship with God, I did notice a pretty extreme difference between her management of loss and mine. In this episode that I watched, the Duggars went to a prenatal appointment where they would hear the heartbeat and find out the sex of their baby, pregnancy number 21. However, when the ultrasound got under-way, it became apparent that the baby was no longer living. I can only imagine the pain that they then went through, as a couple, a family, and a mother. But their first and foremost response was thanks and praise to God for allowing them the time they did have with their unborn child. I'm pretty sure that's not how I would react. In fact, I'm positive.

Let's jump back in time a little bit. Jon and I were in Thompson Falls and I had been tracking my ovulation (or lack thereof) through ovulation prediction kits. Again. I hate those things. Maybe that's just because they never gave me the answer that I wanted. But anyway, I had been tracking my non-ovulation and was so tired and frustrated and felt like God had totally and completely abandoned me. I was a lost soul, and I say that with all honesty and truthfulness. There have been dark times on my road through infertility, but this by far was the darkest and deepest I'd ever been. All my life all I'd ever wanted was to be a mom. I had more baby dolls than you could throw a stick at, and each day growing up, I would imagine my babies that I would one day have and hold in my arms. After about four years of intently trying, without any success or even hope for success, I was becoming severely depressed. I've worked in mental health. Psych is my background and I know the symptoms of depression and I was a walking poster child for Prozac.

If ever I had thought about ending things, it was now. No one seemed to be able to help me. No one understood what I was going through. For all I knew, my God had completely abandoned me. I was done. I climbed into bed that night and started soaking my pillow with tears, begging God to give me an answer as to why this was happening, demanding that he show me what to do, where to go, and to answer my cries. And what do you know, he did. Some people don't believe that God still talks to us. Some don't think that we can still hear his voice, but I'm not some people. I do believe he communicates with us through a variety of things, from the people he puts in our lives to the songs on the radio. That night he didn't just communicate via another source. I heard his voice. I kid you not. Now I know what you're probably thinking: *Sure, Marcy* (insert sarcasm here). *The crazy girl on the brink of madness heard God's voice and not just what she wanted/ needed to hear in her hour of desperation.* Well, you can think that if you want, but I know what I heard, and I heard his voice. It didn't tell me what I wanted to hear. I didn't get the answers to the question I asked. I got the only answer that matters. In that still, calm voice he said to me, "Be still."

To which I responded something along the lines of "Say what?"

"Be still."

But, God! I can't! I need a baby! I want a baby! Why won't you give me a baby?

"Be still and know that I am God."

By now I'm sobbing, my pillow was soaked, my face was riddled with tear stain rivers and I whispered, "But I can't."

He says one more thing, "Trust me."

The funny thing is that a few weeks later in church, our pastor addressed the origins of the verse "Be still and know that I am God." Let me just segue this with our pastor was an incredible pastor. He is the most down to earth, tell-it-like-it-is preacher I've ever met. So when he preached, on his stool, down by the entire congregation and not up on a stage, I tended to listen. Anyway, Bob was talking about this phrase and the origins and translation from the original text to English. It turns out that when read as it would have been in the original context, it's not necessarily the quiet, calming voice that we tend to think of when reading the Psalms. Nope, not so much. Really, when read as originated, it pretty much comes out more like: "Stop your whining and be quiet. Listen to me because I am your father and I know what's best for you." Makes sense to me and seems pretty accurate to the context in which it was given to me. It was time for me to suck it up, to quit being so full of myself, and let go and let God. So see, that seems to be the difference between Michelle and me. She's faced with incomprehensible loss, and she praises God. I need to be told to toughen up, buttercup. Not because my loss is any less, and in many ways I think far greater, but because (contrary to what I'd like to believe) this little world doesn't just revolve around me, and while I don't always understand and likely never will, sometimes I just need to be still.

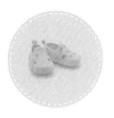

GADGETS

I've done a great many things in my quest to get preggo. One of which is enlisting the help of various gadgets and doohickies to help in knowing when the right time to hit the sheets might be. This has included a long list of ovulatory predictors. Here are the top ones. Ovulation prediction kits: here're seven sticks, go pee on them. Thermometers: check your temp each morning *before* you get up. Yeah, I'm not cognizant of anything prior to that first cup o' joe, so we all know how successful that one was. Calendars: count the days and figure it out. But I think my favorite, just for its lack of any sense and its oddity, had to be the spit kit. Yep, that's right. I don't think that's the actual name. I can't remember what it was really called, but spitting was the basis, so that's how I remember it.

Here's the principle behind it: supposedly when you're ovulating, your body goes through such a major change in hormones and what not that you can even tell the changes in your saliva. To complete this test is quite simple. You purchase a testing mechanism (I found mine on clearance at Walmart) that is a small cylinder-shaped object about three inches tall and one inch wide. Removing the cover will reveal a small piece of glass with a light beneath it, which is activated by pushing a small button on the bottom of the cylinder. Then, as is pretty self-explanatory, you place a small drop of saliva on the glass slide and wait for the sample to dry. In other words, you spit on some glass and wait for it to dry. Once it's dry, you press the little button and search the slide for a pattern. Yep, you look for a picture in your spit. If you are indeed ovulating, the pattern on the slide formed from your saliva will look like fern leaves, thus called "ferning." If you're ferning, it is an optimal time to try and get pregnant.

Lord have mercy, just thinking about it makes me laugh. Ironically, I was always ferning. Shows you how well that worked!

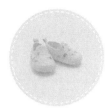

THE PAPER PREGNANCY

It had become pretty obvious that I needed a break from trying to get pregnant. I felt like a hormonal, hot-flashing pincushion. To make matters worse, I was feeling rather alone in the whole situation as Jon had never taken in a sperm sample for evaluation. So in October of 2007, I made a decision that I had hoped not to make for many years. I decided to go back on birth control. I needed to be able to have some control over my cycles and, additionally, to wipe out the chance of pregnancy so that I would just stop hoping for a while. I hoped that this would give me the emotional vacation that I so desperately needed. I broke the news to Jon and he said he understood, but was disappointed. I was heartbroken. I reminded him that he had never taken in a sample and that I felt incredibly alone in all of this. When I filled the prescription, I cried. It seemed like giving up, and I had tried for so long and for so hard to get pregnant. I felt like such a failure. My body had failed me in ways that it never should have done. I grieved the loss of never feeling my child move within me, of never bringing a babe home from the hospital to a freshly painted nursery. But there appeared to be nothing I could do about getting pregnant, so it was time to move on, at least for a little bit.

I had always toyed with the idea of adoption from foster care, but it was cemented one night when a segment of the news called

Wednesday's Child aired. The purpose of Wednesday's Child is to bring to awareness how many kids are looking for a forever home and, hopefully, spur a few more people into getting involved with foster care. On this particular evening, the featured child was a beautiful little boy named Samuel. He was only five years old, and my heart was instantly involved. I scribbled down the number and called first thing the next morning. I talked with a very kind woman who told me that I wasn't the only one whose heart was captured by Samuel, but there were some things we would have to do first before we could ever be considered for an adoptive placement. So during the summer of 2007 I began researching foster adoption. I was blown away by how many kids, from toddler to seventeen, were orphaned in our country and surprised to find photo listings of children waiting for their forever family. It seemed to go against every grain of my nursing HIPPA knowledge to put not only names, but pictures of kids in foster care on the Internet. I requested information from the state and we were sent a packet that sat idly on our computer desk for weeks. Finally and at my whit's end, I told him I was done.

"I'm not doing this anymore," I said.

Jon looked at me with a puzzled expression. "Doing what?" he asked.

"Trying to bring us children. I'm not doing it anymore."

"What do you mean?" Jon asked.

"I've done everything. I'm the one who's seen all the different doctors. I'm the one who's been prodded and poked. I'm the one who's gotten all the paperwork and done all the research for adoption. Me. And I'm not doing it anymore. If you want kids, you're going to do it yourself for a while." I handed him the packed for foster-adoption and walked away to cool off. A few days later he had filled out the packet and we sent it to Marie, our county adoption social worker for review.

Soon she was in touch with us and we began the process of becoming licensed as foster parents and completing our home study. Fortunately for us, I knew Marie on a professional level from the children that I work with and we didn't have to build on a stranger-to-stranger relationship. In an effort to become licensed quickly, Jon and I attended the first licensure class we could and found ourselves spending a weekend in Hamilton. It was quite the training, and we learned more about the state's stance on reunification. According to Montana, it's always the best option, regardless of how many chances a parent gets. After the first night of training, Jon and I needed to get out and walk around for a bit, but Hamilton is a pretty small town, so we found ourselves wandering through the local K-Mart. I couldn't help it; I went straight for the baby isle. I knew our chances of actually having a baby placed with us for adoption were slim to none, but we were finally in a place where things were moving forward with some certainty. And a girl has got goals, after all! Training wasn't the end of our process and we continued by getting fingerprinted and updating our home to the requirements of the state. Even though we only planned to adopt, you have to be licensed foster parents for the process as there is a six-month trial period after a child is placed in your home until you can finalize. So we bought extinguishers, an astronomical amount of smoke alarms, and gathered letters of reference so we could become parents. The process has been called the "paper pregnancy" and it is aptly named.

While we completed our home study, we would meet with Marie every couple of weeks and discuss our history, our plans for the future, and why we wanted to foster-adopt. She asked us a multitude of questions about our family, how we planned to parent, and what support systems we would have should a child be placed with us. Then one night she asked a question I never thought I would hear. She looked at us both squarely and said, "So are you two over the fact that you won't have kids of your own?"

I'm sorry, can you say that again? Jon and I looked at each other, dumbfounded. Had she really just said what we thought she said? Something so incredibly insensitive, and from a professional family worker at that? Looking back on it, I know that she hadn't meant to be cruel. She truly and honestly didn't think that what she was saying was out of line and she had the best interest of potential children in her heart. But still, we were deeply wounded. No, we were not over the fact that we will never have children, and we never will be. But that doesn't mean we won't be excellent parents to the children in our care.

We continued to try and meet the requirements of foster-adoptive parents. We planned emergency escape routes, and baby proofed the house, just in case. During this time Marie would tell us stories of former adoptive parents she had worked with and discuss with us our expectations. One story she told us was about a couple who waited twelve years for their first placement. Twelve years! Are you kidding me? I thought there were thousands of kids in foster care and looking for a family? This just cemented the reality that in order for us to really have a child placed with us, we needed to advocate for ourselves. That wasn't the only horror story. She also told us of a couple who had battled infertility as well, but had a baby placed with them nearly two years prior. Their adoption had been in process for over a year and now was being repealed by the father who was in prison. What the heck is wrong with this picture?

We cautiously continued. We met with Marie on a consistent basis for interviews together and interviews separate. She asked about drug and alcohol abuse, our families, our jobs, what we would do about day care, and if I would stay home. I told her about a little boy I had found on another adoption website, and she promised to send our information to his social worker.

"I know you guys want a younger child," Marie stated one night as we sat in our living room, sipping hot tea and discussing the future of our family. "But would you be interested in someone a little older?"

Jon and I looked at each other. We knew that getting a younger child as a placement was often very difficult, especially if you didn't foster them for a time before parental rights were terminated. But we also knew that older children tend to come with a lot more issues, and at a grander scale.

"Well," we ventured, "do you have someone in mind?"

"Well, yes and no," she said. "One of our workers in Libby has a little girl named Hannah on his case load. I think she's six, or just turned seven, and has been living with a step-grandma off and on for the last few years."

"Where are her birth parents?" I asked.

"Dad is out of the picture. In Oregon or California, I think. And mom is in a treatment center. I'm not sure about placement. They may have someone in mind, but you two just seem like a good fit. She has a half-sister, Rainey, who lives with her dad, Jason. I know he has shown some interest in adopting her to keep the girls together, but I think he also knows that it would be too much for him to take on. He's said that he loves Hannah, but he needs to be a dad to Rainey too and single parenting is hard enough with one child."

"Well, get us more information," Jon said. "We'll take it from there." After all, you can't tell us a little girl needs a home and not care.

By January we were officially licensed as foster parents and were completely legal to take a child into our home. As excited as we were, it was still such a blow to find out someone was pregnant and we were still where we always were—waiting. We had sent in home studies for four children, but each had been rejected for one reason or another. I think my favorite excuse was for the little boy in Texas. His social worker actually said, "Well, don't they have snow in Montana?" Yep, we sure do. We also have this wonderful invention called a coat. Apparently they don't use those there.

The next few months were a frustrating roller coaster. We would get tidbits on Hannah, and then hear that they had found a placement. Then a few weeks later we would find out that the placement hadn't worked. Then her step-dad was going to adopt her. Then he wasn't. Meanwhile we were still trying to keep our options open and researching other children across the country. It's so hard not to fall in love with these children as you read their stories and ache to hold them in your arms.

One afternoon, during my daily searches of foster-adoption photo sites, I found the profile of two little girls in Oregon. The sisters were both young. Sylvie, the oldest, was eighteen months, and her sister, Brooke, was only nine months old. It was apparent that Brooke had been diagnosed with Down syndrome and a congenital heart disorder, but Jon and I didn't care and I loved them instantly. I e-mailed their social worker and provided him with all of our contact information, as well as a copy of our home study and Marie's information. Then we waited. A couple weeks later, Jon and I were overjoyed to find out that our home study was chosen and we were one of four families who had requested to adopt the girls. We tried our best to be patient and waited a little longer for further news. Over a month passed, and we still had no news. About a week later, I was leaving a meeting for one of my clients when I ran into Marie.

"Did you get my e-mail?" she asked me and my heart leapt at the possibility that we had been chosen. In my heart I'd been decorating our spare bedroom for these little girls for weeks.

"No," I replied, trying to calm my nerves.

"Well, I heard from Oregon. They picked someone else."

I was heartbroken. Again I felt like I had lost my child. And to harden the blow, the news was delivered without a sense of sincerity or concern. When I read my e-mail, the one that was supposed to deliver the news that we would still remain childless, it was a mere two sentences. The same she told me in the hall. This was the beginning of my understanding of working with so many social workers. While that is their job, they often fail to remember that this is our life. Being rejected as parents is a terrible blow. What so many don't realize is that once that home study is submitted, we're in. Jon and I have made the commitment, and as far as we are concerned, we have made the commitment to be that child or children's parents. Telling us we've lost is like a miscarriage, each and every time. No one realizes that. They forget the emotional investment that we've made, and once again, we are back to square one. One my drive home I called my sister in tears.

"They didn't pick us," I said. "For the girls in Oregon. They didn't pick us."

"I'm sorry, Marcy," she said, sadness in her voice. "It just wasn't meant to be."

My dad was outraged. He's not an angry person, and for him to show his displeasure isn't something that happens often. But in our world, you don't mess with the family—especially daddy's little girl.

"What's the matter with them?" he cried in outrage. "You two are smart, educated people. They're making a mistake."

To make matters worse, that evening my Bible study met and we studied the life of Sarah, who God had promised children but she was forced to wait until she was an elderly woman. I tried to keep up a brave face, but I was so lost and broken I just couldn't do it. I don't particularly like becoming emotional in front of other people, but that night I shed more tears with that group of women than I had ever done before. It was one more heartbreak and one more set back.

Jon and I started over, submitting home studies and trying desperately not to get attached to the faces on the computer screen. Finally it got to the point that I couldn't look at the websites anymore or submit home studies. I had felt so rejected too many times, and it just didn't seem to be happening for us on this route either. I felt lost and abandoned, sure that God had forgotten the promise he had made to me. I kept wondering what I had done to make God turn his back on me and my pain. In the mean time, we would get random updates on Hannah. Still waiting for her forever family.

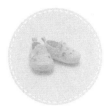

FINDING HOPE

I had an interesting conversation once with a friend. She had children of her own, but was trying to get pregnant again and hadn't been successful. She had miscarried about a year prior and it had taken all of that time for her to conceive again. I'm a pretty strong girl, and I've got a pretty firm faith, though I'll not lie, this experience with infertility has shaken it more than once. Due to these attributes, she confided in me that she was concerned about miscarrying again, which I could understand, but then she made a comment that broke my heart. She said that maybe it was God's will for her to miscarry so that she could suffer, and maybe through that suffering she could be stronger and possibly help others.

Hold up there, honey. I don't think that's how this works. I've been in some pretty dark places along this journey. I've cried out to my maker in pain, I've felt lost and abandoned, and I've wondered if this was a punishment of some sort. But the truth is that I know, with every fiber of my being, that my God, my savior, the lover of my soul does not want me to suffer. Regardless of the pain and gut-wrenching heartache that I have been through, I know that he has cried with me. Does that mean that I like it? Nope. Does that mean that I don't get angry? Not a chance. Does that mean that I don't think this is unfair, unjust, and uncompromising? Sure doesn't.

So what does it mean? Well, I can tell you (as I've said in "What *Not* to Say"), the last thing I want to hear about is how this is his plan. The second to last is to have patience and pray. Right up there with that are the reminders of all the blessings that I do have in my life. Here's why: I'm well aware that I am incredibly blessed in things that many others are not. But you know what? My relationship with God is just that: mine. To me it's like the parable of not trying to pick the speck out of someone else's eye before you pull the plank out of your own. It's not your job to remind me of what I have when all I feel is loss. It's not your job to try and make me feel like I'm lower than you in my faith when all I want to do is curl up in the loving arms of my Father and try to understand why. It's. Not. Your. Job. And it's not helpful; it's hurtful.

Why then, does God allow for these things to happen? And I say *allow* because I believe with the utmost of my being that he does not want or intend, but allows for tragedy. I don't know honestly. I do know that we don't live in a perfect world. I do know that there is pain beyond measure, and we all have burdens to bear and grief to manage. So while I don't know why, I do know that I'm a doer, and this is what I can do. I can create classroom presentations for vulnerable populations that focus on this topic. I can bring awareness to a subject that is considered taboo to discuss, as breast cancer once was (And look where the research and awareness on that is now! My little nursey heart quivers with excitement.). And I can do this, hopefully reaching out to others who have felt this pain. I can pray for guidance, though there will never be understanding. I can pray for peace, when I know that there will always be grieving. Because I do not think he wants us to suffer, I can find hope.

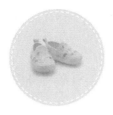

FEAR

There are so many things that are difficult about adoption. Aside from the whole never-getting-pregnant thing, there are new and completely different things that you worry about as a parent. Most people have children and go through the typical concerns and worries: will my child be healthy, how can I help them succeed in school, how can I keep them safe, etc. When you adopt, you take on not only the usual suspects of fear and compound them with a whole new picture of terror. Only a parent who has adopted can truly recognize the terror that grips you at times.

Jon and I toyed with the idea of infant adoption, and we looked into various ways to do this, but there was always one thing that really held us back: fear. Did you know that when you adopt an infant, taking them home from the hospital and signing the paperwork doesn't guarantee that the little bundle of joy you're taking home is yours for keeps? Nope, it doesn't. The birth mother has at least six months, depending on the state, to change her mind. At which point that child that is wholly and surely yours is no longer your child. Regardless of the fact that you have loved, provided, and cared for them. Knowing that the first six months of their life with us would really be a crap shoot, I just couldn't do it. Not to mention the cost of buying a child. There is just so much wrong with that.

And there are so many other unknowns. Depending on the agency you work with, you are likely required to pay the full adoption costs within the first year, even if a child isn't placed with you during that time. And if they do place with you, you have the incurring cost of a newborn on top of the fees associated with the adoption. It's ridiculous. Then there is the issue of whether or not you have an open adoption, and if so how open that adoption is. When we looked into Catholic Social Services, we were surprised to find out that all adoptions were required to be open, and the limitations on contact were not decided by the adoptive parents, but by the birth mother. Some people are okay with this and think it's a beautiful thing, but remember that whole territorial momma bear thing I told you about earlier? Yeah, I'm just not that girl. I don't have any problem sending pictures and keeping a birth mom updated on their progress, but I would so not be comfortable having a birth mother standing over my shoulder questioning or commenting on how I'm raising their child. As far as I'm concerned, once that babe crosses my threshold, it's mine. So there are a few reasons why we never went that route.

But the main reason we chose to adopt from foster care has more to do with the kids and less to do with our fears and expectations. Like I said earlier, when I was in nursing school, I worked at a residential treatment center for young girls. Nearly all of these girls were currently or had been previously foster children. Most of them had no idea where they would be living once their treatment goals were met, and each one of them craved so much for the parents they either never had, or the parents theirs could never be. The home was their family, and those of us who worked there became the big sisters they didn't have or the stand in maternal example they so wanted. It is amazing how quickly you bond with these kids that society and blood have abandoned. Once you learn their stories, you can never be the same. Some of the girls were up for adoption, and it was heart wrenching when they would meet and interview for a placement that would end up not working. One night when we were making rounds, ensuring the girls were all where they were supposed to be and ready for bed, I was telling one of the girls good night and she responded by saying, "Goodnight, Mom." My heart broke and I reminded her that I wasn't her mom, to which she replied that she knew, but wished that I could be. How could their parents cast them off like this? It was so heart breaking and infuriating to see the horrors so many had lived through and the hope they still had for the future.

For most of us, as adults, we recognize when someone acts in a way that is unacceptable and horrendous in our eyes. After this, we typically, unless particularly masochistic, make the decision to learn from the situation and exclude them from our lives. So many people, when they hear about the atrocities that kids in foster care have lived through, assume that the child now recognizes the horrid things their parents did to them and no longer wants them to be a part of their life. That's just not how it works. What we often fail to realize is that the relationship between a parent and child is unlike any other relationship out there. When it all comes down to it, all we really want in life is our mom and dad's love and affection. So regardless of the atrocities their parents may have committed, kids in foster care ultimately still want that parent. They still want them to love them, to say they're sorry, or not—just to be there in general. Because what could make you feel like less of a person or as absolutely unwanted as a parent who does not make the effort to ensure that you are with them? Unfortunately, there are more than four hundred thousand kids in foster care right now. That's nearly half a million kids who are praying for someone to be that parent that they need.

After working at the girl's home, I moved back home to Montana and got a job working as a children's mental health case manager. My new employment opportunity gave me the chance to spend time with multiple kids in my community, and I soon learned that many of the children on my case load were also foster kids, or had been at one point in their lives. While all of my clients occupy a space in my heart, there are two who I hold particularly close. Both had been so neglected by their parents and damaged by the choices their parents had made, and both so desperately wanted parents who would love and care for them.

Due to these experiences, Jon and I decided that with all the kids who needed parents and our strong desire to be parents, adopting from foster care seemed to be a good fit. We had some stipulations though, the biggest being that while we would adopt from foster care, we would not be foster parents in the traditional sense. Getting kids out of the system was our goal, fostering that system was not. If I had learned anything from my work experience, it was that the foster care system is incredibly fractured and breads mental and emotional disorders. The amount of kids in care with diagnosis such as reactive attachment disorder (RAD) is terrifying. With the current state of the system, it's not surprising. After all, in the state's eyes, reunification is always the best option, regardless of the amount of times birth parents are in and out of treatment centers or on various parenting plans. This ultimately results in children pulled from their homes for the first time to be passed to a foster home, back to the parent, back to a new foster home, and maybe a series of foster homes between parent contact. It's no wonder then that a child who enters the system at two and then is finally placed for adoption at seven has some significant attachment issues, along with anger and a whole host of potential emotional disorders including post-traumatic stress disorder (PTSD) and depression. So yes, we would adopt, but we would not be an accomplice to the foster care system.

With that decision made, we had to recognize all of the additional fears of parenthood that would accompany our child. Their birth parents have already proven to be volatile. Could we really protect our children from their further actions? What about other family members? How do we address the reasons that they were adopted without making them feel like they are not as worthy and entitled to a family as any other child? How will our family and friends react to our adoption of a child with potential mental and emotional concerns? What about those mental and emotional concerns? Are Jon and I capable and strong enough to handle the potential difficulties that are rooted in a past we know little to nothing about? The answer to all of these questions was unknown. What we did know was that there are far too many kids in need of a home to let a little fear stand in our way.

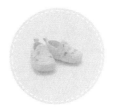

HANNAH

My father-in-law works for a company in Kalispell in which specialty fuel systems and other manufactured parts are made and distributed. One of his employer's major clients is a company based out of Michigan and founded by three incredibly family focused brothers. Each year two of the brothers would make a trip to Kalispell in which they would invite the families of some of their key contacts to join them in a feast of all feasts and a night of getting to know each other. One summer Jon and I happened to be home when this event was taking place, and we were invited to join in the festivities. I was particularly excited because Ken, Jon's dad, had told me about one of the brother's story of adoption. It turns out that though they had biological children, he and his wife had also had a heart for adoption and, as a result, had overcome all the trials and stipulations and had a successful adoption from Russia. I couldn't wait to meet him and chat a bit about their experience.

True to form, the dinner that evening was fantastic, and the company was just as great. Jon (the brother, not my hubby) was more than happy to share his tale, and his pictures just as any proud papa would. He also shared the news that he was in the process of writing a book based on their experiences, and I was so excited to one day receive a copy of the book, with a note of encouragement to Jon and I written on the inside cover. In their story, *The Marvelous Journey Home,* the author tells about how his wife made a book for their adoptive daughters. The book had pictures of their family and special places so that she could keep it with her during their times apart and at least be somewhat familiar with faces when she made her trip home. I love this idea, and when Jon and I started submitting home studies, I compiled my own book. Within it I had pictures of Jon and I and each member of our immediate family. I also included pictures of our nieces and nephews as well as some photos of places we like to hike to and camp at. I thought, if anything, it would be a great representation of who we are, and it would give our potential child a chance to get a bit used to our names and faces before being thrust into our home. When Marie called to tell me that Hannah's social workers had made the decision to place her for adoption, I was ready.

We quickly found out that while parental rights between Hannah and her biological father had been terminated long ago, the rights between her and her biological mother, Tori, hadn't actually been severed until the previous February, only five months prior. The reason for this was fairly complicated. Though Tori had been in and out of treatment centers for the majority of Hannah's seven years (yeah, she was seven, not six), she had also been involved in a relationship in which she and her boyfriend, Jason, had a daughter four years younger than Hannah. As both Tori and Jason had pretty rocky personal lives that often included drug abuse, Jason's mom, Sharron, had stepped up to the plate and taken all four of them in on multiple occasions. As a result, when Tori started spiraling downhill again, Sharron had the responsibility and became licensed as a foster parent. This allowed her to maintain care of Hannah when Tori entered treatment and gave Hannah and her sister, Rainey, the opportunity to stay together. In addition, Jason had become Hannah's pseudo stepfather and she would also stay with him on the weekends on a fairly consistent basis. Due to this multifaceted web of care and the fact that rights between Rainey and Tori had never been terminated, it took quite some time for the decision to finally allow Hannah to be adopted was made.

On July 19, 2008, the meeting for placement was held. We were one of four families, including a great-aunt and great-uncle in New Jersey (who she had never met) that were under consideration. I had given Marie our book in case we were chosen so that Hannah would have the chance to get a feel for us before our first meeting, if we were the family chosen for her.

I was on pins and needles. I didn't have to work and couldn't concentrate long enough on anything to do something useful or creative. By noon, there was still no news.

"I don't know what is going on," Marie said. "I've e-mailed Mike but I haven't heard anything back yet. I'll let you know as soon as I do. I promise."

"I know you will," I said. "I'm really trying to be patient, but I'm not very good at it."

"It's okay. Call me whenever, I really don't mind."

In the mean time, I had talked with my parents, Jon's parents, each of our siblings, and a few close friends, all wanting to know the news.

The next morning Marie called and explained the situation.

"Apparently there have been some legislation changes," she began. "Because there is biological family involved in the process, all permanent placement decisions have to be approved by the head of Family Services. Unfortunately, she's on vacation and won't be back until next Monday."

"Are you kidding!" I asked. "How can they not tell us and make us all wait even longer?"

"I know. I'm so sorry, Marcy. As soon as she's back from vacation, we'll get this straightened out."

Jon was heartbroken when I told him we had to wait another week.

"How can they do this?" he asked.

"I know, babe. That's what I said too."

"Well, I guess we've waited six years. What's a couple more days, huh?"

The thing is, I'm not a patient person. This was my family on the line, and I needed to know if I was going to be a mom or not, so I devised a little plan.

"Hey, Marie, it's Marcy," I said into the phone the next day. "I know you haven't heard anything, but I have a little idea to get us some information."

"Okay," she said. "What's your plan?"

"I think we should call Mike and tell him I want my picture book back. If he says okay, we won't have been chosen. If he says I can't have it back, I think that's a pretty good sign they chose us."

"You're good," Marie said through a chuckle. "So here's the deal, unofficially, you're not getting your book back."

"What!" I exclaimed. "They chose us?"

"They did, but it's not official until it gets signed off, which won't happen until the supervisor gets back. So you can't tell anyone but Jon. All right?"

"All right," I said, my eyes filling. "Thank you so much!"

"You're welcome. Remember, it's not official and there may be a hurdle with the aunt and uncle in the running. But I think you'll be fine. Talk to you when I have the official word."

I couldn't believe it. I was stunned. This was it. I was unofficially a mom! The biggest thing to happen in my life and I couldn't even tell my mom who was coming to visit that day! This was going to be torture!

Jon was ecstatic. "You mean they really chose us?"

"Yep, guess we better paint the back bedroom!"

"Oh my gosh. This is awesome! And I'm scared to death!"

"I know! Me too!"

Jon and I were elated, but we couldn't say a word. Three more days passed and my family called us daily for news. I painstakingly had to keep my big mouth shut. Not an easy task. Even Sharron didn't know what was happening, and she was the one taking care of Hannah. On the other hand, there was always the concern of her relatives in the back of our minds. Sure they were blood, but we had a strong argument on our side. Not only had they never met Hannah, but they also wouldn't be able to keep her in contact with Sharron, who was the only grandmother Hannah had ever known, and her sister Rainey.

The next day I was on a plane headed to training in Salt Lake City, Utah. Jon and I still hadn't received the official word, and I was so disappointed that we would find out and not be together. But there wasn't anything I could do about that at this point. Later that evening I was in a dinner training session when Jon sent me a text: *We got her.* We had both received messages from Marie, though his had come through first. We were semi-parents of a seven-year-old girl we had never met, and we were thrilled.

I called everyone I knew: our parents, siblings, and some close friends. One of my greatest supports during this whole ordeal, from our very first days baby shopping in college to now, was my dear friend, Carol. Not only had I celebrated her pregnancies with her, but she had been a constant support through our foster care battle. Not only was she a loving mom, but she had been a foster child herself and was finally placed in a permanent placement when she was ten. Carol's story is beautiful in that rights with her biological mom had never been severed, and it wasn't until she turned eighteen that she made the conscious decision to take her parents', the ones whom she had lived with and who had loved her, last name. She was thrilled when I told her our news.

Later that night I jumped on a bus with some of my classmates and we took a trip down town. On our ride into Salt Lake, we talked about our backgrounds and eventually our families. For the first time in my life, I was asked if I was a mom and I got to say yes, and then followed it with "well, sort of," and told our story.

Typically parents get nine months to buy the things they need for their soon-to-be babe, and I so wanted to get Hannah something just from us. As I wasted time waiting for my flight home, I scoured the Salt Lake airport for potential things to buy for our first meeting with Hannah. In one of the ridiculously overpriced gift shops, I found the perfect gift. It was a small pink velvet heart that opened to reveal a silver crown necklace with the word *princess* on it. I loved it, but I didn't know if it would be too much, or if I was being silly, so I called (guess who!) my sister and told her of my find.

"Marcy, she's yours," she said after I explained my concerns. "You can get her whatever you want, and she'll love it because it came from you."

Problem solved. So I bought a little pink heart while a little girl in Montana that I had never met singlehandedly stole mine.

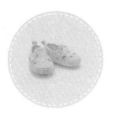

JUNO

Have you ever seen the movie *Juno*? I love that movie. I love Ellen Page's interpretation of her character, and I love, love, love (!) Jennifer Garner's representation of hers (if ever there is a movie made of my life, I want Jen to play me). If you haven't seen it, here's a little rundown: Juno is a high school student who does the deed with her somewhat boyfriend and ends up pregnant. Initially she decides she's going to have an abortion, but changes her mind when she runs into a girl from her school who is protesting outside the clinic. What is it that brings the change of heart? When Juno realizes that her baby has fingernails. Isn't it funny what can change your mind, make something that seems so abstract tangible? But I digress. Juno decides to keep the baby and, making a very adult decision, wants to place the baby for adoption with a couple that she finds through an ad in the newspaper. What results is a somewhat tumultuous relationship between Juno and the adoptive parents, Mark and Vanessa. One of the things that I love most about this movie is that it brings some of the challenges of infertility to light. While we, as a society, tend to play up the wonders and warm and fuzzies of adoption and how wonderful the whole situation is, what gets overlooked is the reality of what the adoptive parents have been through to get to where they are.

At one point in the movie, Juno goes to visit Mark and Vanessa and she finds that there are an abundance of baby things laid out in the living room and Vanessa walks in carrying more. Juno responds with a typically teenage snide comment, but Vanessa responds with the information that a baby shower for them wasn't likely, that they'd been through this before and the birth mom changed her mind. We don't usually hear those stories, do we? The loss that real-life Vanessa's feel is palpable. That's something that people outside infertility don't seem to understand. For us, a loss like that is comparable to a miscarriage. The only difference is that we don't have a physical manifestation of our symptoms—it is all emotional. After all, you can't actually see someone's broken heart, but it's there none the less.

I can relate to that on so many levels. Jon and I have adopted, and we are blessed beyond measure by our three kids, but there are voids that will never be filled, things that we will never experience. Like a baby shower. As you know, we adopted from foster care, which meant that it was (absolute best case scenario) six months before our adoptions were finalized and our kiddos had our last name. It also meant that there wasn't a nine-month build up of preparation. There was no guarantee we would have a child placed with us or how old that child would be. And once we did have our kids placed with us, it was such a different form of becoming a family that most people didn't know how to respond. We, as humans, are uncomfortable with what we don't understand, and for many people, adopting a child who isn't an infant, or going through infertility, is a foreign thing that can't be understood. So regardless of the fact that we were, in all reality new parents, no one ever thought to throw us a baby shower or anything like one. It's not that I wanted the stuff (though let me tell you, double strollers and kid supplies are expensive!), but it would have been really great to have had the experience. Just a little validation that we were becoming parents, taking a huge step, and opening a new chapter in our lives.

So often it feels like people look at us like we're just pretend parents, playing a part because we haven't had all the traditional experiences that come with parenthood. And it's not that we weren't open, with everything. I'm a nurse and I'm pretty straight-forward with everything, so I had no problem talking to people about our struggle. The problem was that no one wanted to listen. Like I said, we don't like to talk about things we're uncomfortable with. So while I'm not uncomfortable talking about it (obviously), others were. Even those close to me, or maybe especially those close to me. It was so frustrating to try and share this huge part of my life with those I love, only to be shut down because they didn't understand what we were going through and as a result didn't know what to say to be supportive. Like Vanessa, things like baby showers would never be part of our baby process.

I think one of the most poignant things about the movie *Juno* was at the end. Vanessa meets her son for the first time and is holding him in the nursery when Juno's stepmom comes in, stopping short at the sight of her. Vanessa asks how she looks, eager to get approval, so wanting to finally look like and be a mom after waiting for so long for that dream to come true. I know how that feels. Wanting so bad to be accepted as a parent.

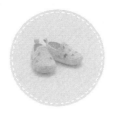

FIRST IMPRESSIONS

It's funny that when you think of entering into motherhood, you are flooded with a mass amount of images related to the task: cuddling in a hospital room while you breathe in that new baby smell or delivering at home, surrounded by your family and friends with soothing music playing in the background. What you don't typically picture about your first meeting with your child is a river raft, cold Montana water, and a picnic, but that's how our first meeting with our soon-to-be child was. After all, she was already seven, and meeting in the labor and delivery room wasn't really an option.

The next couple of days were whirlwinds of e-mails and schedule changes between Marie, Mike, Jon, and I. The goal was to do a slow transition from Hannah's current home to ours, giving us all the chance to get used to each other and promote bonding so that when she did move in, she wouldn't feel so alone or scared. We decided that the first meeting would take place a week after we found out we had been chosen. Mike had the brilliant idea of doing a float trip for the initial interaction as opposed to sitting in an office and trying to get to know each other for the first time. So Jon and I drove to our set pick-up site where we met Mike for the first time. The whole drive to the river Jon and I did everything we could think of to keep our nerves down. There were silly stories of reminiscing, loud country music, but our individual nervous habits still took over and we both fidgeted the full two-hour drive. In our jittery anticipation, we arrived early and were able to spend some time with Mike before Hannah, Sharron, Jason, and Rainey arrived.

Mike is the traditional big teddy bear type of character. His bushy beard and sparkling blues eyes reminded me of the classic mountain-man grandfather we hear so much of in our Big Sky State.

"So ya nervous?" he asked after our initial introductions.

"Very," Jon and I both answered, causing a low chuckle to rumble deep within Mike.

"You know, she's a great kid. I've worked with her for a long time and she doesn't have a lot of the same issues that most of these kids do. Especially for how long she's been in the system," he said.

"It really doesn't seem like it," I replied. "All my experience with these kids and after all the child descriptions we've read, you get pretty good at reading between the lines, and Hannah really didn't seem to have the problems you usually see."

"No, she doesn't. And you guys just really seemed like a good fit. I would recommend that you get together with her therapist, Val, though. It would be good to get her perspective on things too. She and her husband were actually thinking of adopting Hannah at one point and she spent a few weekends with their family."

"What happened?" Jon asked.

"Well, I think a lot of it was just the fact that Hannah is so outgoing, and Val's already got a couple of kids who are both really quiet. It seemed like Hannah may have just overpowered the boys with her social butterfly attitude when they are more introverts."

This poor kid, I thought. *How many families had she been with and houses did she live in thinking that she was finally home only to have it all ripped away from her time after time?*

"Did Hannah know Val was thinking of adopting her?" I asked.

"No, she always just thought she was going for sleepovers. Well, here they are," Mike said as a black pickup pulled into view. "Ready?" he asked, a twinkle in his eye and a grin spread across his face.

"As we'll ever be," I said. Another chuckle from Mike filled the air as we prepared to meet our daughter for the first time.

When she stepped out of the truck, it struck me how beautiful she was. Her dirty-blond hair shone in the hot summer sun and her blue eyes glistened with nerves and anticipation. Sharron and Jason shook Jon and my hand as Mike made the introductions. Hannah stuck close to Sharron and shook our hands with a small smile as we said hello. Her little pixy of a sister wasn't as nervous and helped with the introductions and packing as we loaded everything into the raft in preparation for our trip.

"Hey, Hannah, do you want to ride with Jon and Marcy to the drop point?" Mike asked. "It's only a few miles away."

"Um, sure," she said a little hesitantly and in a small voice. But she seemed pretty confident in her quite demeanor. Jon and I exchanged looks. *Here we go*, we said to each other. *We're about to be alone in the car with our daughter, who we don't know from Adam. Yikes!*

Hannah followed us over to our car, climbed inside, buckled her seatbelt, and sat perfectly still with her little hands folded in her lap. *She's as nervous, if not more, than we are,* I thought.

The short trip to the drop point went pretty well. We tried to make small talk, asking her favorite color—blue, her favorites to do—fish, swim, play. Jon was elated at the fish part. I've never known any one who fishes as much as my husband, and it was always his dream to have a child he could teach to fish and create the memories with his own child that he had created with his dad and grandfather. *Small blessings,* I thought. *You never know what they're going to be.*

At the drop point we all piled into Mike's truck and headed to the loading dock. The girls, Sharron, and Jason squished into the backseat and Jon, Mike, and I filled the front. In this more comfortable environment, Hannah started to open up a little more. We heard all about their trip to Oregon this summer and going to the zoo for the first time, the two girls telling the story in tandem and making us all laugh with their tales of the trip.

The float itself went really well. We all piled into Mike's raft with Hannah, Sharron, Rainey, and myself in the front, Jon and Jason in the rear, and Chris paddling in the middle. Initially Hannah was distant. She kept a good distance between the two of us, and when we brought out the fishing poles, she was determined to do everything herself. But as the trip wore on, she began to inch her way closer to me. Soon she had climbed up to sit on the side of the raft and scooted closer and closer to me. We chatted with Sharron and Rainey and she told me about her school and day care and more about her trip to the zoo. She loved any small rapid Mike took us through and would squeal in delight as we both got drenched from the waves. As thrilled as I was to be learning more about my daughter and building the beginnings of a bond with her, I felt terrible that Jon was stuck in the back and hadn't had a chance to interact with her very much at all.

The longer we floated, the hotter it got as the Montana July sun beat down upon us. The girls were especially toasty as they had the extra bulk of life vests. About halfway down the river, Jon did something unexpected. My normally gets-hypothermia-in-the-bathtub husband said he was going to jump in the river. Mind you, it may be hot outside, but the river was freezing. Hannah's eyes widened as she became giddy with excitement.

"Can I jump in with you?" she exclaimed.

"Sure, I'll catch you," Jon said, and over he went.

As soon as his head surfaced, Hannah jumped into the river with him. They both gasped in shock at the temperature and we quickly pulled the goose bump–ridden two back into the raft. As they gained their breath back, they both started laughing, and we all teased them for being crazy enough to dive in. But Jon's plan had worked. The ice was broken, and before long, she went to join him in the back of the boat and of her own volition.

Before we knew it, we were at the pick-up point and climbing out of the raft. While Jon and Mike drove back to pick up the other vehicle at the launch point, Hannah and Rainey played in the river, becoming increasingly brave as their bodies numbed to the frigid water. This distraction gave Sharron and I the first opportunity to really talk.

"She seems like a great kid," I said.

"She really is. She's dealt with a lot because of Tori and, amazingly enough, has come through things really well." Sharon's tone dropped and her face became somber. "Tori is not a good person," she said. "She and her mom both are really into drugs and alcohol, and Hannah got caught in the middle of it. She's been with me off and on for the last few years. Jason, Tori, and the girls moved in when Tori got pregnant, and they were in and out for the next few years. I tried to help, but then they would mess things up so much in my life I would kick them out. Pretty soon they'd be back though. I couldn't let the girls live the life Tori and Jason were living." Now I was really learning some of the reasons Hannah was placed in care to begin with, and it was heart wrenching. I couldn't imagine letting this beautiful little girl go through the terror of a drug-addicted care giver. I can only imagine the things she saw in her little life, and how frightened she must have been.

"But you need to know that you guys are her family now," Sharron continued. "She has no one. We'll want to stay in touch of course, but she doesn't have grandparents, aunts and uncles, or cousins. No one whom she knows and is appropriate for her to be around. You guys are it. That's why I'm so glad they chose you. Now she can have a ton of family that really support and love her."

"We're so excited that she is going to join our family, and so is every one else. Our parents and siblings can't wait to meet her,"

Marcy Hanson

I said. "They've been with us through this whole process and are ecstatic to have another little girl joining our family."

"Did Mike tell you what she said when she found out about you guys?" Sharron asked and I shook my head no.

"Oh." She laughed. "It was really cute. I went to pick her up from day care and Mike had come to see her already and give her your book. When she came out of the building, she was so exited and said, 'Grandma, did you hear the news?' I had of course, but wanted to let her tell me her exciting news so I told her I hadn't. 'They found me a family!' she said. It was so cute, and she was so excited." I felt my eyes welling with tears and was thankful I still had my sunglasses on.

About that time Jon and Mike returned and we had to coax the girls out of the water. Though we hadn't really touched before, Hannah took my hand to help her out of the water and, under the guise of play, gave me my first hug, soaking me with the chilly water of the river. As she climbed back into our car to go do dinner, Rainey shocked us all by asking to ride with us too.

"You two okay with that?" Mike asked.

"Sure," Jon said. "The more the merrier.

The trip to the restaurant was filled with the girls' laughter and stories. Hannah interpreted for us a number of times as Rainey still had the high-pitched little girl voice that is often unintelligible except for close family and friends. When we reached our destination, Jon and I began getting the girls out of the car.

"You two look pretty natural at that," Mike said with a grin. "How's it feel?"

"Pretty natural," Jon replied with a smile and we headed into the restaurant.

Dinner was a combination of chatter, keeping the girls entertained, and nervous silence. Fortunately there wasn't a whole lot of the latter. At one point, a woman who none of us seemed to know approached our table and started talking to Hannah and playing with her hair.

"Who are you?" Rainey demanded.

"I'm one of Hannah's grandmas," she replied, which only baffled us more. "Which makes me your grandma too because I'm really Jessica's grandma."

At this point Mike was looking at her like she was crazy, Jason and Sharron looked genuinely confused, and Jon and I were getting pretty uncomfortable with the fact that this seemingly stranger was touching our daughter's head and calling herself grandma. Just as I was about to ask her to leave or explain herself, Hannah surprised us all. Obviously uneasy with the situation, she got up from her chair and instead of going to Sharron, what I think we all expected, she came and stood between Jon and I and put her hands and chin on my shoulder. *She must really be okay with this after all,* I thought, and the crazy old lady that no one seemed to know finally left.

After dinner we made our good-byes, and Jon and I climbed back into the car for our drive back to Thompson Falls.

"What do you think?" I asked as we pulled out onto the highway.

"She's great," he said. "And Sharron is great too. I think it's pretty impressive that she stepped up and took Hannah in when she didn't have to."

"Yeah, I know. She filled me in a bit on Tori. Sounds like she was the one who made sure Hannah was safe most of the time."

"Really? How so?"

"Well, I guess she went over to Tori and Hannah's apartment a couple of times when Tori and Jason were broken up. Hannah didn't have a winter coat, or a bed, or even blankets to keep her warm. Sharron went back and made sure she had a coat, then got a hold of a friend of hers who is a quilter, and was able to get Hannah a warm quilt for nighttime."

"That just pisses me off," Jon replied. "Not Sharron, but that Tori would allow, that any parent would allow their child to live like that. Jason doesn't seem like a real winner either."

"I don't think so either. Did you smell the pot that seemed to waft off him and his car? I didn't like seeing Hannah climbing into it. He seems pretty high strung. Like ADD to the max."

"Yes, he does. I'm not a fan. And it kills me a little each time she calls him dad."

The rest of our trip we rehashed all the little details. There seemed to be so many similarities between the three of us, and it became apparent that though we had first met, Jon and I were head over heels for that little girl. We couldn't wait to spend more time with her and were so disappointed that things hadn't moved quicker as in a couple of days we were headed to a family reunion and all we would be able to take of our little girl were her pictures. As soon as we got home, I ran into town with my flash drive and started selecting pictures of our meeting with Hannah to print. Okay, maybe I printed all of them, but hey, I was a new mom, remember? I was amazed when I got them back. While I realized when we first met that there were similarities between how she looked and the two of us, that realization was compounded when the pictures were developed. One shot of her and Jon showed just their profiles, which were darn near identical. The same went for facial expressions. She had the same look or smile as one of us on multiple occasions.

Those pictures became my new best friend. They went with me everywhere. We took them to the family reunion, where everyone was amazed at our similarities. I took them to work and pulled them out each time a patient asked if I was a mom or not. I showered all of our friends and acquaintances with the photo proof that we really were going to finally be parents. And each night we talked with Hannah on the phone. While we knew we needed to take things slow and not push anything, it was so hard not to jump right in. I wanted to tell her I loved her, and I couldn't wait until she finally called me mom.

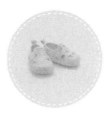

MAKING CHANGES

Though we weren't able to see her again, we did call Hannah and talked for quite a while each time. She would tell us about her day at day care and give us play-by-plays of whatever she happened to be watching on TV. When we said we couldn't wait to see her again, our hearts lifted when she replied, "Me too." When I talked to Sharon she said that Hannah had really enjoyed the weekend and that she sleeps with the picture book every night. "She sleeps with that book you made her every night, and she wipes it clean every day so it doesn't get ruined." My heart ached, such a sweet heart and spirit this little girl has, and to be waiting for a family when she should have been secure in a loving home to begin with. I could only imagine the stress and worry that had filled her little mind, wondering if she would ever have a forever family.

For our next visit we again drove to Libby and this time rented a hotel room. Mike, Sharron, Jason, and the girls met us there for dinner, and then we all headed to the pool where we played for hours. It was an excellent way for us to build trust with Hannah as she would jump into the pool and we would catch or teach her tricks in the water. After a bit, everyone else left and Jon, Hannah, and I had our first opportunity to spend some time alone. We played in the pool a bit longer and then we all went up to the hotel room to dry off and relax for a bit before we took Hannah back to Sharron's house. Jon and I sat on the bed and we all chatted and watched cartoons. Before long Hannah had climbed up with us and cuddled in to watch TV. We were both surprised at this initial show of comfort and affection, and I don't think any of us wanted the evening to end.

The next morning we met every one again for breakfast, and afterward, Mike, Sharron, and Hannah joined Jon and me on a short hike nearby. We had a wonderful time in the woods. Jon helped her skip rocks, we played in the sand, and we threw sticks off a swinging bridge. As it got closer to the time to leave, the normally chatty Hannah became more subdued. But she had good reason. This time when our visit was over, she wasn't going back to Sharron's. She was going to come home and stay the night for the first time. As we started home she barely spoke at all, and Jon and I were concerned she was too overwhelmed. After all, she didn't know us that well and now she was coming all the way to our house and stay the night. How much can a seven-year-old handle?

"Are you kind of nervous to come to our house?" I asked. "It's okay if you are. I know I would be."

"No," she replied, looking out the window. "I've been adopted four times before."

I thought my heart was going to break. Had no one explained to her the difference of adoption and foster care? How could she have thought she was going to be adopted before? And what damage was done to her poor little self-confidence? I glanced at Jon, and he seemed to be thinking the same thing, his eyes glazed with tears as mine were.

"Well," I said, "what do you thing about this time being the last time?"

"That would be good," she said.

"Sweetheart, this *is* the last time. We want to be your forever family and have you for a really long time."

She looked at me now, a small, nervous smile creeping across her face and hope, the tiniest glimmer of hope, shining in her eyes.

That evening went well. She absolutely loved playing with our dogs, the golden retriever puppy Moose, and our sweet little mutt Ruby. She and Moose galloped around the house and she laughed wholeheartedly as he tried to lick her to death.

In the morning, I fixed her favorite breakfast of french toast and she gobbled it up like she hadn't eaten in days. Then we talked about how she was going to have her own room and we thought that for it to really feel like hers, we should paint and decorate it how she wanted. After all, it was her room forever, so she should like it and feel at home in it. After searching the Internet for different ideas, she decided what she wanted—polka dots. I had never seen a room painted in polka dots, and Jon looked at me as if to say, "Are you serious? You're actually going to let her paint polka dots?" But we had made her a promise that she could paint her room however she wanted it. So if she wanted polka dots, a spotted room she would have. After all, it's just paint, right?

So off we went to the paint store where she picked her colors—pink, blue, purple, and green. While we waited for them to mix we gathered all the other painting supplies we would need to finish the job. At home we cut out stencils from poster board and lay plastic over the hardwood floors. Then I cut circles out of sponges and we went to work! Not long into our project, Jon's parents, Ken and Linda, stopped by the house. They were on their way to a camping trip and we encouraged them to come meet their grand-daughter for the first time. When they saw what we were up to, they donned some paint clothes and joined in the fun. I'm still not sure who was the biggest instigator, the seven-year-old Hannah or her fifty-something grandma. My bets are still on Grandma.

When we had finished the paining, her room looked surprisingly cute. The colors were adorable and the varying sizes of dots added character. It had turned into such a wonderful weekend, and none of us could wait for the next week to pass so we could see each other again. Our phone conversations in the interim became longer and longer, nearing an hour most times. She was taking a beading class and was really enjoying the creations she was learning to make and couldn't wait to show us her talent when she came back.

The following Thursday, Sharron dropped her at our house and brought with her a few of Hannah's things to make her room more homey and start the moving process. Hannah was excited to show us all her things and give us each surprises; she had made us gifts in the beading class she was taking! The very first necklace she made she wanted me to have, and I was honored to wear it. For Jon she made a beaded frog, which went to a place of display with our family photos. She was so proud to see that we appreciated her gifts. Here, a child with so little, but so willing to give.

The next day my parents were able to stop by and we had a great time going to lunch together, and Hannah seemed to take to them right away also, just as she had with Ken and Linda. On Saturday we went to a local festival where we ate nachos and got snow cones and tried not to melt in the hot August sun. Hannah also had a chance to see a little of what Jon does as his company had a trailer set up with an aquarium and various forms of fish identification. As she peered into the fish tank, the local newspaper photographer snapped a picture of us and asked me what my daughter's name was. Hannah gladly gave her name, and on the way home, I asked her what she thought about being called our daughter. She nodded her head yes. Yes! Yes!

"Would you like us to introduce you as our daughter from now on?" I asked.

"Yeah!" she replied. So here we were, our makeshift little family, still growing and learning, but a family none the less.

After church on Sunday, we decided to have a relaxing day. After all, it's got to be pretty wearing on a child to go through as much as she is and meet all these new people who are now supposed to be her family. So in the afternoon, we took a little walk and stopped at the school near our house to play on the equipment. When it was time to go, Hannah decided she would test and see how far the limits could be pushed in our little family and refused to leave.

"Let's go home, it's time," Jon and I said repeatedly as she continued to slide and kick off her shoes.

"It's time to go home, we're leaving," I said as Jon and I started walking up the hill toward home. After a few feet we turned around to see if she was following. There she sat, shoes off and feet dangling off the edge of the slide, not budging.

"I knew you wouldn't *really* leave me," she said in the snottiest seven-year-old voice she could muster.

"I am leaving right now," I said. "Let's go." And I turned and continued up the hill. She slipped her shoes on and caught up with us at the top of the little hill next to the road. Initially she was quiet, but after a minute, she grabbed my hand and walked beside me.

"I've got something in my eyes," she cried and I looked down to see little tears filling her blue eyes.

"Oh, I'm sorry," I said. "That's the bummer about the play-ground. It gets dusty and then you get stuff in your eyes, huh?" She nodded her head yes.

"As soon as we get home I'll put some drops in your eyes to make it feel better, okay?" I said, and she agreed.

When we got back to the house, I sat her on the counter in the bathroom and put a couple drops in each of her eyes. Then I made her look at me.

"We will never ever leave you for good. Okay? I promise," I said, and she grabbed me around the waist and started sobbing.

"We love you very, very much. And nothing can ever change that. We aren't going any where and want to be your forever family." She continued to cry as her tears soaked through my shirt. Jon walked by the bathroom and, seeing us there, came and put his arms around us both.

I continued, "I know it's probably hard to believe that this is for good, because I think you've been told that before." She nodded her head yes.

"Know how I know it's for good?" I asked and she shook her head no through her tears.

"Because Jon and I prayed for a very, very long time for God to bring us a little girl, and he promised us he would, and he brought us you. And God doesn't break his promises." At this she began an all-out sob again, and Jon and I rocked her until the crying ended. When she did stop, I leaned down to look at her and said, "No matter how mad I make you or you make us, we're in this for good, and no one is going anywhere, okay?"

"Okay." She smiled and hugged us again. Over the top of her head, Jon and I exchanged glances. We knew there would be outbursts—it was only a matter of time. There was no doubt in either of our minds that this needed to happen and was a huge great step in the right direction. However, that didn't mean that each time it happened we wouldn't be emotionally exhausted. That day in the bathroom I realized just how much this little girl was going to break my heart.

When it was time for Hannah to go, we loaded her into our car and headed out to meet her grandma. Though Jon and I knew we had made progress that day, we weren't sure how much Hannah understood that or how she would handle the situation as she processed it more. But as she would prove to do repeatedly, she amazed us once again as on the quiet country road she said out of the blue, "Today, I had a really good day."

That week, as we waited for her to come home for good the following weekend, we talked nearly every night before she went to bed. And one night, when we said good-bye and we loved her, she said she loved us too. We had waited so long to be parents, and it was so beautiful to have a child who seemed to feel the same about us as we felt about her.

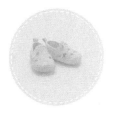

HOME FOR GOOD

On August 15, 2008, our daughter came home for good. Jon and I had both taken leaves from work to provide as much time for bonding and family building as we could before school started—and we had a lot of family building planned. During one of the transition visits, Hannah had mentioned that she had never been to a fair. Fortunately, our hometown county fair was the week after she moved in. We decided that it was a perfect opportunity to take Hannah home with us and have her meet some of her new family. So we called Jon's sister Michelle and told her of our fair plans and asked her to join us. What could be more fun than meeting your aunt while riding the rides at the fairgrounds? Michelle couldn't have agreed more, and before we knew it, we were searching for parking and headed to the dusty grounds.

Hannah and Michelle took to each other instantly. Jon and I had commented before on how similar in personality the two were, and before we knew it, Mom and Dad had taken a backseat to cool Aunt Michelle. The two of them were inseparable, and though she would often check to make sure we were present, Hannah seemed pretty comfortable with Michelle. In fact, I'm not sure how many rides she actually rode with Jon and me. There were of course the activities like mazes and big rides that were done in a group, but anything two seated was reserved for

Hannah and Aunt Michelle. Until, that is, we braved the Starship Trooper. Or as our family lovingly refers to it, the Starship Puker. It was another two-person ride and Hannah and Michelle, Jon and I got into our respective bench seats to endure a spinning adventure. What we hadn't anticipated was just how spinney the adventure was going to be. About five seconds into the ride, I felt sick. Not just normal sick either. Mouth-watering, jaw-tingling, if-they-don't-stop-this-right-now-I'm-going-to-lose-all-the-food-I've-ever-eaten-over-all-of-the-passengers sick. Two words: not good. When the ride finally ended, I slipped my wobbly self out of the seat and kissed the ground beneath me.

"Honey," Jon said tentatively. "You look kind of green. Are you okay?"

"Sick, gonna be sick," I said, searching for all the garbage cans in the close vicinity.

"Hannah doesn't look so good either," Jon stated as we looked to see she and Michelle pouring themselves out of their seats. Hannah was walking at an angle and moaning softly. When she located Jon and me, she weaved her way towards us and heaved her body against mine for support. I don't like getting sick, I don't think anyone in their right mind does, and I rarely vomit. But when I am sick to my stomach, I don't want to be touched—by any one. Yet here I was, locating trash cans like a GPS navigational system and rubbing the back of my little girl who looked slightly greenish herself.

The rest of the weekend was a whirlwind of family. It's amazing the change in dynamic your life takes with your own parents when you yourself become a parent. Linda was thoroughly enjoying not being the one to scold and correct for things like table manners, that is, "Hannah, we eat our spaghetti with a fork, not our fingers" was now my job to say. When she wanted to go for her first motorcycle ride on my dad's bike, my father told her she had to ask her parents and said to me, "It's up to you, honey." Suddenly I wasn't just a big girl anymore. I was a mom. Holy crap.

Though we tried to do some school shopping, most of our weekend was spent getting to know family as Hannah met some cousins and aunts and uncles. So the following week, she and I took a day to go shopping. A few months prior, Jon and I had bought a new car, one big enough to hold our expanding family and make trips in. But we still hadn't sold our little Nissan Sentra, an amazingly economical vehicle, and though we had bought and filled out a For Sale sign, hadn't really made up our mind if we were going to sell or not. As there was no reason for Hannah and me to take the big car, we climbed into the Sentra for our little school shopping road trip. In the backseat, Hannah found the For Sale sign and asked me about it. I explained that we were thinking of selling it, but hadn't really decided yet. I thought nothing of the sign until a few miles down the road when I glanced in the rearview mirror and saw Hannah flashing the sign to all passing vehicles.

"That truck driver looked at me funny," she said as she raised the sign in anticipation of another passing car.

Chuckling, I thought to myself, *I can't imagine why*. About an hour into our trip, she asked if we were almost to our destination.

"My arm is tired," she explained.

"You don't have to hold that sign, silly girl," I replied.

"Uh-huh I do. That's my job." Matter of fact and all, the kid has spirit.

The following weekend, we had a small family reunion of sorts on Flathead Lake. My brother Tim and his wife, June, children Kendall and Claire were all camping on the lake so we all went to join them. Hannah was going to meet almost all of her cousins on my side, quite a feat since I'm the youngest of five and have twelve nieces and nephews. The only ones missing would be my sister Mindy and her family as they had recently moved to Pennsylvania.

Hannah had a blast. She and Claire took to each other immediately, and being the only little girls there, who could blame them? But Hannah had a great time with the boys as well. Kendall, only a year younger than Hannah, took to informing the younger cousins, James and David, four and two, about Hannah.

"That's your new cousin Hannah," he informed James in his husky in-charge voice.

"I know," replied the younger cousin.

"She's almost eight," Kendall replied.

"She's getting big," James responded. And the two left the verifications and acceptance at that. She's our cousin, and she's getting big. What else mattered?

The following Monday I got my daughter ready for her first day of school. Rather a surreal feeling, if I do say so myself. On our school shopping spree, we had found the most adorable dress with black, white, and green swirls. She had also gotten black leggings and dress shoes and we had arranged the outfit the night before so she was all prepared. She walked out of her bedroom the next morning in the dress and leggings, a little black sweater, and what-was-this socks in her pretty back dress shoes. Not just any socks. They couldn't have been black or even dark blue so as not to be so noticeable. Nope, they were light brown with various shades of pink flowers on them. Now, I understand a fashion statement, and I also understand the fragile workings of a little girl trying to look her best and rather grown up. So I approached the subject with caution.

"Hannah, why are you wearing socks with your leggings?" I asked tentatively.

"My feet were cold." Bless her and her practicalities. What can I say? When your feet are cold, you put on socks. Even if you're wearing a dress and leggings.

Her first day of school went well. She and her teacher got along splendidly and she seemed to enjoy her classmates. We were off to a good start. The next day, things were a little different. I had to drop some paperwork off at the school, and Nurse Judy, the school nurse and a friend of mine, approached me.

"Can I talk to you for a minute?" she asked.

"Sure," I said, giving her the hug we always exchanged.

"Hannah came to see me today," she said, her voice slightly concerned.

"Was she sick?"

"No," Judy hesitated. "She got bit."

"Bit?" I asked. I could feel my momma bear claws coming out. "Who bit her?"

"A little boy in her class. It didn't break the skin and I cleaned it well. She's fine but I wanted you to know."

I could feel my face heating. Someone bit my child? "What happened?" I asked.

"I don't really know, but I wanted to tell you."

I thanked her and went to join Jon in the car.

"She was bit today," I said and together we tried to figure out why on earth someone would have bitten our daughter. When we picked her up, she climbed into the car all smiles.

"How was your day?" I asked.

"Good!" she replied.

"I hear you got bit," I said. Her face crumpled and her pale skin became red and blotchy, with tears forming at her eyes.

"What happened?" I asked.

"Logan bit my arm," she replied. We know Jeffery. He lives across the street from us and has a less than normal home life.

"Why did Jeffery bite your arm?"

She shrugged her shoulders.

"What was happening when he bit you?" Jon asked.

"We were playing on the playground."

"And he just bit you?" I inquired. She nodded her head.

"Did you say anything to him?" And she began crying, silent tears as she pulled a mangled piece of paper out of her backpack. It was a letter from the principal. Dear Lord, second day of school and we're getting a note from the principal. This doesn't bode well for the future. The page stated that she had been teasing him and he had bitten her. So we asked what she had teased him about.

"I was saying he had a girlfriend," she explained.

"Why?" we asked, and she shrugged her shoulders. By the time we made it home she was a weepy, blotchy mess. We all went to the kitchen table and discussed the matter more.

"How does it feel when people tease you?" I asked.

"Not good," she replied in a tiny voice. "But Ms. Green said that Logan was in more trouble because he bit me."

"Well," Jon said, "we don't agree."

"It's wrong to bite someone and hurt their body," I said. "But words can hurt a whole lot more than anything else. We have to be very careful with our words. No matter who we're talking to."

"What is your punishment for school?" Jon asked.

"You guys have to sign this paper and I have to take it back to Ms. Green," Hannah said.

We signed it and asked Hannah to go get a blank piece of writing paper.

"Now you need to write Jeffery a letter telling him you're sorry," I said.

"Okay," she said in a quiet voice. Behind her tears, there was the underline of fear in her eyes.

After she finished the letter, we stapled it to the note for her principal and put it in her bag for the following day.

"Hannah," I said, pulling her chin up to look me in the eyes. "We love you. Even though you got in trouble at school today, we love you and that will never change. No matter how much trouble you get into, we love you." She grabbed us around the neck and burst into tears. Jon and I looked at each other, wariness and concern in our eyes. We'll make it, we said to the other's heart. We'll make it.

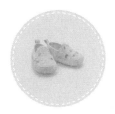

HANNAH'S IMMA

The seasons were finally beginning to change. The air had become crisp with autumn's glory and the leaves began to take on their brilliant hues of red, orange, and yellow. School was in full swing and going pretty well for Hannah, who had now been with us for a month. We had definitely grown as a family. She expressed often how happy she was that we were adopting her, how much she loves us, and was constantly cuddling, on our lap, and finding any way to be close both physically and emotionally. Not to mention she wrote our last name as hers on everything she owned with no coaxing from us.

At this point, the only step she had not made to become a full-fledged part of our family was calling us mom and dad. We were still Jon and Marcy, though there had been some progress in her referrals to her birth and stepfamily. Her birth mother had become "my mom Tori," her stepdad was now "my dad Jason," and so on when it had once just been "my mom and dad." Still, every time she referred to Jon or me by our first name, it was like a knife through my heart. For so long we had waited to be parents, and so long I had wanted to be a mom, in every sense of the word. Though the actions and everything that I did represented "mother," the title, and perhaps what made it seem most real, was denied me. No matter how much I rationalized that she had only been with us a month and she's had a hard life, etc., etc., I still so longed to be called mom and felt like an impostor trying to play the part without the title.

Especially when it seemed like every one I knew was asking, "So has she called you mom yet?"

Petty, I know, but until you've been in my shoes, I don't think you can ever understand. We had mentioned in small ways that we would like to be her mom and dad. On walks we would wish on dandelions, and Jon and I had both told her we wished that she would call us by our parental names. She would grin, grab our hands, and continue on. But still, she would only say it by accident. It was obvious how badly she wanted to call us mom and dad, but refused to let herself have the liberty. I knew there were so many issues that could be playing a part in her decision, from uncertainty of the permanency of our family, to the fact that in the past "mom and dad" hadn't necessarily been good things, so why pass that on to us?

I tried to gain understanding directly from the source, Hannah. We were chatting one day and I nonchalantly asked her if people at school ask about our situation.

"Some do," she said. "But not many people."

"What do you tell them about our family?" I replied.

"Well"—her eyes lit up—"I tell them that you're a nurse and you help people, and that Jon works with fish."

"What do you call us at school?"

"Jon and Marcy," she replied. My heart sank some. Perhaps, I had thought, perhaps she calls us mom and dad at school, and just not at home. There went that hope.

"When people ask you who your mom and dad is, what do you tell them?" I inquired. At this point the conversation was still very light. She's a very open child and really willing to talk about pretty much everything.

"I tell them it's you guys." Well, here's a little move in the right direction.

"How do you feel about calling us mom and dad?" I asked.

"I don't want to." Insert knife and cut out my heart here, after all, now it's broken.

"Can you tell me why you don't want to?"

"I just don't," she responded.

"Do you not think we're your mom and dad?" I asked.

"No, I know you are," she replied. Well, that's something.

"Do you think it's going to hurt someone's feelings if you do?" No response.

"It won't," I continued. "Your Grandma Sharon, Dad Jason, and Mom Tori all want you to be happy. They know that you're being adopted and in another family but that you will always be part of their family too, and nothing can change that. So it's OK to call us mom and dad when you're ready."

That was the end to our conversation at that point. I tried to hold back my tears at the fact that she just flat out didn't want to call me mom and move on.

But my heart hurt. I tried to seek out support and guidance in this area. The last thing I would do is force her to call me mom. After all, hasn't most of her life been forced to do this, do that, live here? Let's put some stability in her life and withhold the guilt. I turned to my friends first. I received the standard response: It'll come, give it time. Time. Time. Time. I'd given it six years. Didn't any one understand my feelings and perspective? In all their attempts to be supportive, it didn't quite hit the mark and often made me feel worse. One dear friend even tried to comfort me by saying her daughter didn't call her mom for nearly a year. True enough, but slightly different when the child can't talk in the first place and you've given birth to her. I think another thing that people often failed to realized that when she didn't call me mom, it broke my heart, but when those around me didn't refer to me as mom either, the insult only went deeper. I told Jon at one point that I was going to send a mass e-mail to every person I ever met requesting that they refer to us as mom and dad to Hannah so that at least someone would acknowledge the fact that we are raising this child.

My next step to gain support was to reach out to the online community of foster-adoptive parents that I had become a part of. I logged on and made my first post. The body of my piece explained our battles with infertility, the time we've waited during the placement process, and how thankful I am for the little girl living in the polka-dot room. Then I explained my feelings about being called mom. I expressed that I knew it would take time, probably lots of time, and I knew that, was trying my best to be patient, but it really hurts to go through the motions and not get the name, and was there any one out there who could understand and offer some encouragement? What I received shocked me. While my post expressed my rationalization of my emotions and asked for support, the responses were, for the most part, anything but supportive. Instead I was told that I have no right to feel the way I do, after all, it's the child who has lead the horrible life, and that I had not waited long enough to deserve being called mother. I was shocked. I was horrified. I was hurt. The community who was supposed to understand, who had dealt with what I have, who was not like the general public who had no idea why we would ever adopt an eight-year-old had turned on me. If I could not turn to them, who could I turn to?

Jon was right there with me of course. He wanted to be dad as much as I wanted to be mom; he just didn't dwell on it as much as I did. But we gave it time. Neither of us broached the subject again for another month or so. Then one Sunday Jon and Hannah were cuddling on the couch talking and he said how much he would like it if she called him dad. He got the same response I did—she doesn't want to. No explanation, just that.

By this time in our relationship building, she had become very secure with us. Her slips of calling us mom and dad had become more frequent and her true stubbornness had come out in full force. She had been testing us the last couple of weeks and was a worthy match to my own stubborn streak. So after the most recent mom/dad conversation, Jon and I began to discuss what we really thought the issue was. Hannah talked openly about Tori, showed us her letters, and even said she didn't miss her because she hadn't seen her for a long time and "I only miss the people that I used to see a lot, like my sister." She had said. So it didn't seem a loyalty or replacement issue. Then Jon made an interesting point.

"I think it's just her stubbornness," he said. "She knows we really want her to call us mom and dad, and this is her way of controlling us. She's being stubborn."

Hmm. Good point. I had previously asked a friend of mine, a former retired army colonel who had adopted two teenage sisters what they had done about the whole mom/dad issue.

"They called me dad from the beginning," he said. "When we brought them home, I told them they could call me Mr. Hill, colonel, or dad. They chose dad."

I had told Jon about this earlier and we started talking about doing this with Hannah. If she's being stubborn, then it's a matter of respect, and even if she's not just stubborn, it was still a matter of respect to us. I began searching for different ways to say mom and dad. I researched various languages in an effort to find something that we would like and would have meaning for us in some way also. I have a very spiritual background and really wanted to incorporate that into my search. What I found and really liked was the name *Imma*, the Hebrew term for mother, and *Abba*, the Hebrew term for father.

Over the next few days Jon and I discussed what we were going to do. Should we propose this new plan, giving her three choices of things she could call us? Should we just wait and let her decided (which very likely could be never)? Or do we wait until everything is finalized and at that point say, "Okay, we're your parents legally and all, so now you have to call us mom and dad"? None of those options sounded particularly appealing. The last thing we wanted to do was force her to call us mom and dad, but if something didn't change, I was likely to lose my mind. And in a hurry.

During a visit from my mom, we started to talk about the issue at hand. She too had wondered if it was just Hannah being stubborn, but also agreed with my notion that perhaps Hannah didn't want to put a label on us that hadn't been so great in the past. If that was the issue, I didn't want her to use the traditional *mom* name either.

"Maybe you should talk to her about what it means to be a family," my mom said. "There is no doubt in my mind that she thinks of you two as mom and dad. That's just obvious in her actions. Like a couple weeks ago when you guys were home. She was playing in the playroom with the cousins, but would come out every few minutes just to love on one of you. It seemed very unconscious. She just wanted to know you were near."

"I know she thinks of us as her parents, but it's still so frustrating when she calls us Jon and Marcy. She loves it when we call her our daughter—she's told me so. And she really loves knowing she's part of this family. She has no problem calling you guys or Jon's parents "Grandma and Grandpa" or any of the aunts and uncles or cousins. It's just the two of us that she refuses to give a family name," I said.

"Well," continued my mom, "talk with her about how it feels to be called your daughter and that your family is made up of all the parts, not just a daughter and two adults."

That night I decided to try my mom's approach. We were getting ready for dinner, one of Hannah's favorite times, especially when she gets to help.

"So, Hannah, what do you like best about being in our family?" I asked.

"Well," she started, "I really like how much time I get to spend with you guys, and that we live here. And..." She paused. "I really like that we have pets. Because I didn't really get to have pets before and I really like that we do." Ah, the truth of a child.

"Do you still like it when we call you our daughter?"

"Yeah!" she replied.

"What is it you like about us calling you our daughter?" I inquired.

"I dunno. It just makes me feel good," she said.

"We really like calling you our daughter too. We waited for a very long time for God to make us parents, and so we're really happy you're with us and our daughter too," I said. This brought big grins.

I continued, "It sure would feel a lot different if we just introduced you as 'that girl who lives with us,' huh?" She nodded.

"Probably wouldn't feel very good. Not at all like we're a family, would it?" She shook her head no.

"I don't think it would either. See, that's kind of how Dad and I feel when you call us Jon and Marcy." Now I had her attention. "For us we want our family to have parents and kids, and when you call us Jon and Marcy, it kind of feels like we're just those people you live with."

"There's lots of ways to say a name," I continued. "Sometimes we don't want to call someone a certain name because it reminds us of something else that maybe we don't want to think of with that person. Like when Dad and I talked about having kids. I really liked the name Nathan, but Dad knew someone before who had that name, and he wasn't a very nice person. So every time Dad hears the name Nathan, he thinks of him, and we didn't want to give our son a name that brings back bad memories. And there's lots of different ways to say mom and dad. We just wanted to think about that a little, and how we want to be a family, in every way possible."

"Okay!" she said, and we continued dinner.

After our meal and during cleanup, I decided to subtly bring up the issue again while in a totally different manner that was unrelated to her actually calling me mom. First though, a little background information. During the first few years of trying to conceive, I was very hopeful. I had faith that the promises God had given me to make me a mother would indeed come true. Jon and I had always talked about getting tattoos, but we wanted to do something that was really meaningful to each of us, as it would be permanently on our bodies and all. We thought it should be more than some random ink. At twenty-five, I had decided. I designed a piece with a stargazer lily, some ribbons, and the word *hope* in the Greek language spelled out beneath the flower. To me, it is very symbolic. Not only is the lily my favorite flower, Christ was also called the Lily of the Valley. I wanted the word *hope* not only for the hope and knowledge that God would follow through on his promise, but for it to be in Greek, a language of Christ.

All right, back to Hannah. As we were putting away the dishes and clearing the table, I told Jon I was thinking of adding on to my tattoo. Instantly interested, Hannah perked up.

"What are you going to do?" she asked.

"Well, I was thinking of putting the word *Imma* below the word *hope*," I said.

"What does that mean?" she inquired.

"*Imma* is the Hebrew word for mother."

At this her face lit up, and my quick husband interjected, "You could call her Imma if you wanted."

I continued, "See, the word *hope* represents the hope that I had that one day God would make me a mom, and he did! It's written in Greek because that's one of the languages Jesus spoke, and I would like *mom* in Hebrew because that is another language Jesus spoke and it's very special to me." At this she threw her arms around me in a tight hug and huge smile.

Soon after I had to leave for a meeting, and by the time I returned home, Hannah was in bed.

"Guess what we did all night?" Jon asked with a smile.

"What?" I replied.

"After you left, she asked me how to say *mom* in Hebrew again. I couldn't remember exactly so we looked it up and found *Imma*. Then she wanted to look up *dad* in Hebrew, *Abba*, and *daughter*, *Bot*, and *sister*, *Achot*. She thought it was really cool. Even wrote *Imma* and *Abba* on a piece of paper and taped it to the mirror in the bathroom because she said she'd probably forget again."

As per ritual, I went into her room to kiss her good night, and in her state of absolute sleep, she batted me away like a distraction. Not unusual to get an odd response instead of waking when she's pretty much out cold. The week before, in the same situation, she had sat straight up in bed, looked at me, and told me I was just a dream before falling back on her pillow.

The next morning Hannah came and cuddled with me for a bit before getting ready for school.

"Did I push you last night when you came to say good night?" she asked, laughter in her voice.

"You sure did," I told her.

She giggled and said, "I can't believe I pushed Imma!" My heart leapt.

"Guess what!" she continued. "My name is Hebrew! And so is Jon's! And *Abba* means 'dad,' and I'm Bot! And I can't remember the name for *sister*."

"We can look it up," I said.

"Nope. I wrote it on a piece of paper and put it on my wall, 'cause I'm tricky, tricky!" she said.

So here we were our little English family with Hebrew names. Another language or not, she had finally called me mom.

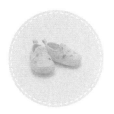

CONTACT

As a foster-adoptive parent, one must endure a six month "trial period" until the adoption is finalized. Basically, we're all on probation to make sure it works. I can understand this theory. From what I've learned, other states require a much longer time frame, up to nearly two years in some cases. Six months is hard enough, in my opinion. Here's what happens: you become a child's parent. You take them to school, prepare their food, wash their clothes, comfort their bad dreams and fears, you do all the parenting things. Then you ask for permission. You ask permission to take them on trips to see their grandparents. You ask permission for them to stay the night at a friend's house, to take them hunting, and probably a whole mess of other things that quite frankly slip my mind. After all, I'm the parent, right? Wrong. On a technicality, sure. But as a foster-adoptive parent, you are constantly reminded that, in all legalities, the child is on loan to you from the state. In case we all change our minds.

Then after asking permission, you are told how to be a parent. You are told when to take them to the dentist and the doctor. You're told to be sure to write thank-you notes to the family who remembered long enough that this child should belong to them to send a birthday card. You are told to keep up the contact with the child's birth family. Fortunately for Jon and I, our social worker knows us well enough to allow us to be parents, but there are still the legal aspects that always haunt you until those final papers are signed, sealed, and delivered. Until the time, you parent under the rulings of the state. During this time, it is encouraged that the child remains in contact with the birth family. This helps the child establish and maintain their roots. It is also a roller coaster of emotions for all involved. Often after a visit with birth family or even a phone call or letter, the child is thrown into an emotional upheaval that can take days or weeks to recover from.

But we understand the importance of these relationships and felt it important to keep Hannah in touch with her birth family. Rainey was a definitive part of Hannah's life, and would therefore remain in contact. We encouraged at least weekly phone calls and participated in visits. For Halloween, I took Hannah to her hometown to carve pumpkins with Rainey. They had a great time, aside from the fact that Rainey was feeling under the weather and they ended up spending a good portion of the day cuddled together watching cartoons. Jon and I prepared ourselves for the tantrums to follow, but to our astonishment, they didn't come.

Instead, Hannah told me on our way home, "I'm glad we went to see my sister. I really miss her." Then when we reached our house, she climbed up on Jon's lap in the living room and told him, "It's good to be home." What an amazing blessing. We had expected the worst, but our little girl was glad to be home. That's not to say that all contact has come with bright smiles and a lack of emotional turmoil, quite the opposite.

We were particularly amazed after Rainey spent the weekend with us a couple months before we finalized. With the holiday season well upon us, we had been trying to get the girls together for a visit, and while Hannah wouldn't be leaving our sight, we welcomed her sister to our home. When circumstances allowed, Rainey came to stay the night one Saturday. Sharron dropped her at our house early in the day and promised to return on Sunday. The girls were thrilled to see each other. So much so that neither even told Sharron good-bye; they were already playing in Hannah's room. Jon and I had been a little apprehensive about the whole visit. After all, what we knew of Rainey was that, though a sweet girl, she has the potential to be a handful. We were concerned how events would play out, and that Hannah would fall back into the "mother" role and breaking her free of that again would take some time. Not to mention the huge emotional turmoil of having her sister with her constantly again, only to leave one more time. Prayers for peace in all situations were constantly on our lips the whole weekend.

Because we wanted to make it a memorable and fun weekend for the two of them, we had planned to go get our Christmas tree with Rainey in tow and then let the girls decorate it. Of course, being a Montana winter, we woke up Saturday to our first snow fall of the season—six inches and a balmy six degrees. Yikes. But I had asked Sharron to pack warm snow clothes for Rainey and she had. So we bundled the kids and ourselves up, loaded the dogs and all of us in the car, and headed out to find our Christmas tree. Despite the bitter cold, the girls had a wonderful time. They wrestled in the snow, we pulled them on sleds, and they took the opportunity to tackle Jon and me whenever possible. Within a couple of hours their, cheeks were rosy with cold and we settled on some hot cocoa while making our way home. We spent the rest of the afternoon decorating the tree, watching movies, and reading stories. It was painfully obvious how much Rainey wanted a mom and dad, a typical family where life focused on the kids, not the parent's desires. Soon, likely because Hannah was doing it, Rainey began calling us Abba and Imma.

"You're calling them mom and dad," Hannah said with a laugh. But that didn't stop Rainey. She continued to call us both Jon and Marcy and Abba and Imma the whole weekend. At one point in the mid-afternoon as Rainey became sleepy, she curled her tired little body up to me on the couch. I asked Hannah if she would like to come cuddle also. She smiled and declined, but within minutes, she was up on my lap, curled into me as much as she could.

"Pretend I'm your baby," Hannah said.

"You are my baby," I responded.

"No, like a newborn," she replied and cuddled down into my arms like an infant would. When I told Jon of the incident later his eyes got teary and he commented on the fact that she had likely never had that before.

Later on in the evening, Jon played Santa Clause for the girls and they climbed up in his lap to tell them their wishes. At one point in the play session, someone commented on Rainey's nose.

"It's my momma's nose," she said. "My mom. *Our* mom, Hannah. Our *real* mom!" she said with accusation of betrayal in her voice. Hannah sat quiet, choosing not to comment. At four, it had to be impossible for Rainey to understand the situation. She knew that Hannah had a new set of parents, with a new house and room, but she still had the same Grandma, and nothing different had happened to Tori in Rainey's mind. It's a hard concept for an adult to grasp, and Rainey was definitely confused. Aside from the confusion and possible sense of betrayal, the girls had a wonderful weekend. By Sunday afternoon things in our household were back to normal. We had plenty to do to not only get ready for Christmas, but were also neck high in household projects as well. We were planning on refinishing our hardwood floors that winter and Jon went to work at prepping the back bedroom. Soon Hannah had was following him around and asking to help.

"It was nice to have my sister here," she said. "But I feel like I haven't seen you all weekend, Abba." With that, they spent the rest of the day sanding and vacuuming, father and daughter.

After phone conversations with Rainey and Jason, Hannah would often take on the voice and role of the adult, as she had done when living with them. Sometimes it would take quite a while for her to slip back in to the role of child. The more comfortable she got with us, the more she would question the ethics of Jason. Within the first week of her moving in, she would ask if we thought something was right and give us a situation.

For example, on a trip to visit family, she called out from the backseat, "Do you think it's right that you should have to clean up other people's messes?"

"Well, not normally. Is there something specific that you're thinking of?" Jon asked.

"My dad Jason, whenever I would go over to his house, I would have to clean Rainey's room, and I wasn't even there to make the mess. I don't think that's fair."

"In our house, we all help each other, but we're responsible for our own messes too," I said.

"Yeah. I like that. Whenever Rainey hurt herself, my dad Jason said it was my fault too. He said since I'm the big sister, it's always my fault, even if I'm not there. Do you think that's right?"

"No, we don't do that in our house either," I said.

"He doesn't even pay his own rent," she continued. "My grandma pays it, and his food too 'cause he sells his food stamps. I don't think that's right either."

Jon and I were stunned. We knew the situation wasn't the best at Jason's, but we hadn't realized how hard it was on Hannah. We could only imagine what the money the food stamps went too, and we had a good idea it lead to the smell of marijuana that always lingered so close to Jason.

When she received money for her birthday, Jon and I encouraged her to open a savings account so she could put some money away for vacations or save up for something she really wanted. She was far from sold on the idea. We both chalked it up to her age, but continued to encourage the idea. One day after I recommended it, she said that she had an account once.

"You did?" I asked.

"Yep. But I don't have it anymore," she replied.

"Why not?" I asked. "Did you use all the money you saved? Or closed it because you were moving here?"

"No, my dad Jason took it all."

"What do you mean?" I asked.

Her little face became outraged. "He said he needed some money, so he went and took it out of my savings account. Then he never paid me back. Do you think that's right?"

"Not at all," I said. "Money that's yours is just that, yours. We would never take it from you." That seemed to satisfy her, and when she told my mom the story, to which the reply was

"You're mom and dad have their own money. They wouldn't take yours." She seemed more at ease to open her own account. Of course, by then she had spent most of the money on things I had planned to buy her for Christmas, but what can you do? The more comfortable Hannah became with us, the more we learned about her life with Jason. Once when working with Jon she confided that she doesn't like to be alone.

"What do you mean?" he asked.

"Like if Imma is down in the basement and I'm upstairs, I don't like that."

"No?"

"No. I used to be alone a lot. My dad Jason and Rainey would go to the store or something and they would leave me at home or make me stay in the car. And sometimes they would be gone for a long time."

"Well, we're not going to leave you anywhere," Jon replied. To which he received a grin and a hug.

Not long after that, Hannah came in to our room in the wee hours due to a nightmare.

"What did you dream?" I asked.

Her teary voice responded, "I dreamed I was in the car with you and the dogs at Grandma and Grandpa's house and I opened the door and Ruby and I got out and you didn't know, and you left me."

"What do you think would happen if that really did happen?" I asked.

She shrugged her shoulders. "I would turn right around and come back," I said. "I'm never going to leave you." It broke my heart to know that while she seemed to feel secure with us, her fear of abandonment still haunted her.

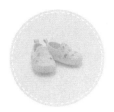

LETTERS

While we continued to hear stories about Jason, Hannah continued to receive monthly letters from Tori. Most were insignificant one or two sentence pages that left Hannah obviously unimpressed. In November, she received one slightly different. It was still only a few sentences. Tori thanked us for the Halloween picture we sent and then wrote one line that would throw Hannah into a loop of loss and pain.

"I'm glad you have someone to do your makeup," she wrote. "I worry about things like that."

Two sentences. Not much by anyone's standards, but two that, for the first time in who knows how long, actually showed some motherly concern. Two sentences that superficially focused on Hannah while twisted back around to center on Tori at the same time. That evening was heart wrenching. Hannah was tender and bruised emotionally and easily frustrated with anything she tried to do. Repeatedly I asked her to talk with me, to tell me how she was feeling and what she was thinking, to let her emotions out so that she didn't bottle them inside. Finally, as we tucked her into bed she broke.

"I just wish I could see her." She sobbed. "I haven't seen her in a long time."

"Do you think things would be different if you saw her?" I asked.

"Uh-huh." She nodded, her face reddened and tear streaked.

"How would they be different?" I quietly asked through tears of my own I refused to shed until I was out of her bedroom.

"I don't know."

"Do you think things would be different here? Like not with us?" I pressed.

"No," she said and enveloped us in soggy hugs.

In the kitchen I broke down, crying into Jon's shoulder, staining his shirt with my mascara.

"Talk to me, baby," he pleaded.

"I don't know if I can to do this," I said. "It just breaks my heart to know that in her perfect world, we don't even exist."

For the first time, Tori had written Jon and me a letter as well. It wasn't very long and was written in the girlish loops that her handwriting possessed. In it, she thanked us. She stated that she had been speaking to Jason and he said how happy Hannah is, and that she was glad to know Hannah was doing well. She also asked if she could send tape-recordings of herself reading stories and talking to Hannah. Jon and I both felt this was a poor idea and would only serve to confuse Hannah and cause her more pain. Marie agreed.

After she received her letter, Hannah was distant for the next couple of days. Tori had sent a coloring picture to her in the letter, and when Jon suggested she color it and we could send it back, she haughtily replied, "I'm going to."

The interesting thing with Hannah is how she processes things. She may be instantly excited or outraged or whatever, but over time, she mulls things over and over in her mind until they make full sense to her. About a week after the letter arrived, she asked me if I was going to help at school on Mother's Day.

"Well, Mother's Day is on Sunday, so you won't have school that day," I replied.

"But are you going to help like before? Because you can't come in right before because then you'll know what you're getting for Mother's Day!" She grinned at me.

Over the next few days, she made similar comments all in reference to different occasions. Then one afternoon, I came home from work and was changing out of my business attire when I noticed something shining on my bed stand. Upon closer examination I realized that the glimmer came from two small rings, charms for a necklace. One was silver with the word *mother* engraved around it, and the other gold with blue stones on the edges. The gold piece had *December* engraved on one side and *love* on the other. I was touched to find these, but refused to accept them as gifts to me at this point. After all, Hannah loved to cuddle in our bed and she tended to leave her belongings all over the house, typical of any eight-year-old. When she got home from school, I hesitantly approached her.

"Hannah," I said presenting the charms, "I found these by my bed this afternoon."

"Yeah, they're for you," she replied and I felt tears come to my eyes. Not one to let her true emotions shine through, she finished with "After all, I'm not a mother, you are."

In early December, Marie came for a visit with Hannah and brought with her Tori's most recent letter. Unlike her normal after-school visits, Marie had come in the evening in order to spend some time with not only Hannah, but Jon and myself as well. When it was time for Hannah to reluctantly take her evening bath, Marie presented Jon and me with the letter.

"You might not want to give her this one yet," stated Marie. "Read it and then decide."

The card itself was standard Christmas: merry tidings and what not, but inside she had addressed it to the three of us and signed it, "Love Tori, the other mom." It was a little surprising and bittersweet to see her signature and self-title, but that wasn't the reason not to share the card with Hannah. With the letter she had enclosed a two-page poem she had written for Hannah. As I read her writing, my heart broke. The poem was all the things that a daughter is—from sunlight to butterfly kisses, and all the things a mother wishes for her—happy days and someone to dry your tears when you cry. The loss I felt for Tori surprised me. I could, in effect, understand what she was going through. Each time I thought I was pregnant and then wasn't, I grieved the loss of a child. This woman was losing her child, day by day for the last six years. At one end of the spectrum, I was grieving for her and the pain she surely was feeling. At the other end, I didn't pity her in the least. After all, she had been given ample time and opportunity to clean things up and regain her daughter. But she hadn't. That was a choice she made over and over again and one that I could never offer her empathy for. I could understand on a cognitive level that this woman had not had a stellar childhood herself, but I'm a firm believer that character is not just something that you're born with, but something you create within yourself.

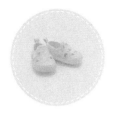

BREAKTHROUGH

O ne of the first things that Jon and I learned about Hannah is that her patience level was pretty low, and it didn't take much to throw her over the edge into a frustrated tantrum. One of the most curious things is that she would often get mad when doing something she's done a thousand times before, but has decided that for this moment it's too hard. Take homework time for example. In the beginning of the school year, Hannah would throw a tizzy fit the size of Texas each night while doing her evening homework. She would pull at her hair, hit the table, stomp her feet, and carry on in all other manners that a two-year-old would do in response to frustration.

"It's too hard! I can't do this!" was the constant response to any task that she may have to think on for more than two seconds or that she had never attempted before. Soon that phrase became outlawed from our house. It quickly got to the point that knots would form in my stomach at the thought of her homework time in anticipation of the battles that would likely follow. Time-outs were instigated and time limits were set on tasks to ensure her work would get done.

One night at Bible study, my group of ladies and I were talking about failure and how we had been raised to handle our lack of successes. During this time Jon and I were dealing nearly nightly with tantrums and time-outs, both of us frustrated beyond our limits.

"In my family," I began, "you just didn't fail. If something didn't work, you tried again. If it still didn't work, you looked at other options to the solution, and if you still had trouble, you asked for help. It was a constant learning experience and failure wasn't an option. You tried and kept trying until you succeeded. It may not always be the first time, but that didn't matter. So right now, with my eight-year-old whom I haven't had eight years to mold, things are rather difficult."

I continued to explain about the near-nightly tantrums and how we were trying to teach her about success and trying again and sticking to something even though it feels hard.

"Well, you're raising a two-year-old," one of my friends stated. "You haven't had eight years to work with her and now you're going through all the developmental stages that you would with a birth child, just at a faster pace. So she may be eight, but in your relationship, she's two."

"Well, my two-year-old knows a whole lot more words that most two-year-olds do!" I replied with a chuckle. We continued to talk about our children, the struggles they have, and how they tend to throw those tantrums at the most inopportune times, that is, isle two of Harvest Foods. As the evening progressed an e-mail was shared about a mother of four who had received a book from a good friend who had recently traveled the globe. This care-free business woman was not burdened down by a husband and children, soccer games and ballet, and the mother of four was beginning to wonder if they could relate to anything at all anymore, especially when she realized the book she was given was on medieval cathedrals. Puzzled she opened the book to the inscription written by her globe-trotting friend, which explained that the book focused on the fact that these wonders of architecture were never built in the span of one man's lifetime and often the original visionary would never see the full beauty of his creation—much like the work of a mother. One section went on to describe a man surveying the work of a cathedral. As he walked through the growing creation, he noticed a carpenter high up on scaffolding, carving a small bird into a support beam. The man asked what the carpenter was doing wasting his time. After all no one would ever see his handiwork. The carpenter replied that he would always know the bird was there; after all, isn't that what really matters?

"See, Marcy," said one of the women, "you're just building a cathedral."

"Honey," I replied, "right now I'm carving a bird."

As time passed, the tantrums became less frequent. She began to learn that though in the past throwing a tantrum meant she wouldn't have to continue whatever task it was that she didn't want, this was not the case in our house. Having a tantrum just meant it took longer to accomplish the task that she didn't want to do.

When the snow began to fly and temperatures dropped, Jon and I began feeling the urge to ice-skate. Hannah showed an interest also and for weeks we talked about how fun it is to ice-skate, but that it is something that takes much practice, lots of falls and bruises, and that it's not a sport that is mastered at once. Over Thanksgiving break, we braved the ice and took her for the first time. The rink was perfect, the ice like glass, and all-around perfect conditions. So we donned our skates and ventured to the ice, her excitement bubbling in tune with our anxiety over the potential disaster that we were anticipating to take place. After all, history had proven that if Hannah was not instantly perfect at her new task, she was more than mad.

The first trip around the ice she fell repeatedly, clung to the rink, gave us looks that could kill, pouted, and by the time we reached the bench, was in the process of beginning an all-out tantrum. Jon and I took a deep breath and began the job of trying to encourage our deaf-with-frustration daughter.

"You're doing great," Jon said.

"You really are. Remember, we said that ice-skating is hard and takes lots of practice." She fumed, arms crossed tightly over her chest, eyes hard as rocks and unblinking, cheeks reddened with rage.

"Did you think you were going to be perfect on the first try?" I asked. No response.

"All right," Jon said. "Let's go. Are you going to join us, Hannah?"

"You have a choice to make," I said, standing. "You can choose to have fun, or you can choose to be miserable."

Miracle of miracles, she got up. She took Jon's hand and started for the ice. We got about a quarter of the way around the rink when a little boy, not older than four, came over to us with an aluminum apparatus designed to steady the beginning ice-skater while they learned how to get their balance on skates.

"Would you like to use this?" My angel in a red snowsuit and lace-up skates asked. I could have kissed him.

"Sure," Hannah said and took the tool. From then on, she was unstoppable. She gained her balance and with that her confidence and began tearing around the rink at break-neck speed. Soon she was skating on her own, unassisted and doing remarkably well. At one point she fell really hard, striking her head on the ice. I know I would have had an instant headache and thought to myself that this was probably the end to our escapade, and rightly so. To our astonishment, she denied even a break, jumped up, and began skating again. Not a tear was shed. Throughout the evening and again in the car on our way home Jon and I showered her with accolades. How proud we are, what an excellent job she had done, that she didn't give up, etc.

"I was sitting on that bench," she said, "and I kept thinking 'This is too hard. I don't want to do this. I can't do this.' Then I decided to have fun and to try again and told myself that I can do it, and I did really good!"

Hallelujah, she was getting it! She had made a cognitive decision to have fun, and it paid off. From that point on, ice-skating was our go-to defense. When she started to protest and things got "too hard," we brought up her ice-skating success, and for the most part, it worked. That's not to say we never had melt-downs again. However, the interesting thing was that often if we caught her early on in the tantrum and told her that she wasn't allowed to throw a fit, she would stop. Or if we began a task with the clear-cut boundaries that a temper tantrum would not be permitted, she would accomplish the feat without a problem. It is amazing how early she had mastered the poison of manipulation and breaking that power was a difficult task. Often I wondered if I was strong enough to do it. But as they say, we are never given more than that which we can bear.

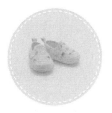

HANSON'S FIRST FAMILY CHRISTMAS

When Hannah joined our family, I was ecstatic at the thought of finally having a child at Christmas time, though it certainly wasn't the "first Christmas" I had pictured in my head over all those years. After all, there were no cute little onesies professing the child's initial year of festivities, no buying ornaments with "baby's first Christmas" embossed in beautiful letters on a cloud supporting a sleeping infant. But I was trying to see passed these things. Obviously my list of firsts as a mother were far from the norm. Why shouldn't the holidays be the same? In some ways it was more fun that what I imagined the infant holiday to be. After all, Hannah could frost cookies; a baby isn't so skilled with baking. So I set out to engross her in all the traditions of my childhood that I could muster. We baked sugar cookies, which she thanked me for making the dough as she'd never made sugar cookies before. She helped me stir fudge and we decorated the house with bows and berries. All the while I subtly tried to build the foundation of why we celebrate Christmas, the birth of our savior.

As my eyes filled with tears over the little drummer boy, I explained humility and the blessing it is that Christ came for each one of us and as a fragile and vulnerable baby. I told her of my childhood family traditions. How every Christmas Eve my family would gather after dinner and my dad would read us the Christmas story from our ancient family Bible. Then we would do Communion together, join hands, and pray for all the things we were thankful for and blessed with over the last year, and all those we hoped for in the year to come.

Of course, we had plenty of fun with the present part of Christmas too. Hannah had asked for ice skates, pink specifically, and only days before we had ordered just that for her. We talked about how wonderful handmade gifts are as I secretly crochet her a scarf and our mothers and sister-in-law prepared homemade gifts as well. Soon she was teasing us about the gifts she herself was making, and each visit we had with Jon's mom, they would escape into a room for privacy to work on gifts for us. After which she would taunt us with the knowledge of what was to come. Like any child, she wasn't so gifted at the actual secret-keeping aspect. After a shopping trip she and I made to buy cologne for Jon, we returned home and she promptly told him we had gotten him a gift.

"I'll give you one hint," she said as I tried to intervene, but not soon enough. She thrust her arm under his nose and proclaimed, "Smell me!"

Jon looked at me and smiled. "Thanks for the cologne, love," he said. Note to self, don't take the eight-year-old Christmas shopping.

Amidst all the holiday hustle and bustle was Hannah's school Christmas concert. For weeks before the event we had been hearing various renditions of the carols they would perform and as the time grew closer, she got more excited. The night of the concert she dressed in one of her favorite holiday gowns, a velvet maroon dress with flowers that sparkled along the bottom.

"Imma?" she said as she hesitantly approached me with her performance attire. "Would you curl my hair for tonight?"

"I think we can probably do that," I replied and was rewarded with an ear-to-ear smile.

"No one has ever curled my hair for a concert before." She babbled as the iron heated and I began sectioning out her locks. She was giddy with excitement as I curled and clipped and I repeatedly batted her fingers away from her head so she wouldn't inadvertently burn herself on the iron. As I finished, she gingerly touched the curls, careful not to displace any.

"Oh, Imma," she crooned as she felt her hair. "Thank you!" My heart warmed and I looked up to see Jon standing in the doorway, feeling the same thing.

The concert was adorable and though her class sang just two songs, Hannah made them memorable. While her classmates stood awkwardly still on stage, Hannah was moving and grooving to the music. After the performance, Jon and I found her giddy and missing her hair clips.

"What happened to the clips I put in your hair?" I asked.

"They were bothering me, so I took them out," she replied. "Well, really I just wanted to see if I could make my curls bounce on stage. Did they?"

"Oh, they bounced all right," Jon said.

Jon and I both laughed, how perfectly Hannah, our little drama queen superstar.

A couple days before the holiday, Sharron stopped by our house to drop off some presents for Hannah. In the bag of gifts were also a few pictures and ornaments, including one with the year of Hannah's birth. I may not have bought it, but we did have a first Christmas ornament to hang on our tree. Small blessings.

On Christmas Eve, we gathered at Ken and Linda's for dinner and festivities. We made and decorated cookies for Santa, and I read to the family the Christmas story before we tucked the anxious Hannah into bed with the direction that she couldn't get up until six. I myself have never been one who is able to sleep Christmas Eve and woke many times throughout the night.

At 5:51 a.m., Jon turned to me and said, "She's got nine agonizing minutes left."

So we waited, and we waited, and she never came. By seven he rolled over to me and said, "You must have been really tired. I've never seen you sleep in this late on Christmas."

"I know, and I can't believe Hannah isn't up yet!" With that we crawled out of bed, greeted Merry Christmases to Ken, Linda, and Uncle Steve, and gathered round the coffee pot. When Hannah still didn't rise, I couldn't handle it any longer.

"Let's go wake her up," I said. Jon looked at me with laughter in his eyes.

"Can't handle it, can you?"

"Nope. Let's go." With that we ambushed her air mattress and woke the bleary-eyed little girl who we had expected to wake us. When she realized what was happening, she was quick to get up and join the festivities. The morning was a blur of wrapping paper and bows. Hannah loved her ice skates and the other presents she had received and couldn't wait for us to open the gifts from her. At her anxious encouragement, Jon and I opened them together. She had made each of us pencil holders for work. They were, however, a far cry from the simple creations I had made for my own parents in childhood. Jon's had water paper background, pictures of the two of them fishing, and various three-dimensional fishing stickers. Mine was covered in nursing memorabilia from 3-D stickers of pills and stethoscopes, to a lap coat with my head and hands glued to it. They were incredibly creative and intricate. Later Linda remarked that everything was Hannah's idea and her only contribution was hot glue. Jon and I each hugged and thanked her, and when our eyes met, each shimmered back tears.

"You have another one from me and Abba," Hannah said, handing me a small package. "You're going to love it, I know you are." She was squirming with excitement as I began to peal back the wrapping paper. Inside was a blue shirt, with *Imma* painted on the bottom right side and back left shoulder. Again I felt the moistness of tears in my eyes.

"It's beautiful, Hannah," I said and enveloped her with a hug.

"Try it on!" she begged. It was a perfect fit, and the pride in her eyes spread to her whole body and she glowed.

That afternoon we went to my parents' house. In my family, baby Jesus isn't put into the nativity until Christmas day and only after we sing him happy birthday. As tradition mandates, he is placed by the newest or youngest member of the family. This year it was Hannah's turn and she took to the task proudly. We had one more present for her at my mom and dad's, the scarf that I had made her. She looked at it and said that it was neat, the kind of yarn she really liked and good colors.

"Imma, made that for you," Jon told her.

Her eyes widened. "You did?" she exclaimed. "How?" "I crochet it," I replied. At that moment she put it round her neck and has scarcely been without it since telling all who comment on it that her mom made it for her.

When we tucked her in that night she was dreary with exhaustion from all the excitement, but one thing was pressing on her mind.

"Imma, when do we do that thing where we all sit around the table and pray?"

"Oh, well, remember when I said that my family hasn't done that in a long time because we all grew up and got married and weren't together on Christmas Eve? That's something we did when I was little."

"Oh," she said. "I was really looking forward to that."

"We can do it right now," Jon said. So we joined hands and began praying. I started and thanked God for the opportunity he gave me to be a mom and for giving me Jon and Hannah, and the wonderful family he has blessed me with. Jon followed suit, and when it came to Hannah, she became teary and thanked God for her family and blessing her too. Such big words and understanding for such a little girl. Though it may not have been the first Christmas I had anticipated, it was so much better than I could have hoped for.

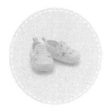

THE SUN
WILL COME OUT

W e made it through the holidays and were on the home-
stretch toward finalization. February 15 would officially
be our six-month mark and we were hoping to sign the papers
as close to then as possible. We weren't the only ones on count-
down—Hannah was numbering the days as well. Inevitably, on
the fifteenth of each month, she would remind us of how close
we were to reaching our six-month date. As excited as we all
were to finalize, we also understood the importance of reminding
Hannah that since we weren't in control of all the paperwork, it
may take a little longer than exactly six months.

"I know," she would say. But the secret hope of finalizing on
the fifteenth was evident in her eyes.

With each monthly visit of Marie, her tension toward finalizing would become more evident. We knew that seeing the social
worker would be traumatic for her, and each time we would deal
with the manifested behaviors of the visit for longer. Marie's
January visit was especially difficult for Hannah. The visit was
rocky from the very beginning. About twenty minutes after school
ended, I received a call from the elementary school secretary.

"Marcy? Hi, this is Donna at the school."

"Hi, Donna, what's up?" I asked.

"Well, I have Hannah here and she thinks she's supposed to go home with Marie today, but she's not here."

"I'll be right there," I replied and headed for the school while trying to reach Marie. I left a message on her voicemail, reminding her of the visit and stated that I would be back home in a few minutes after I picked up Hannah.

There was a message waiting for me when Hannah and I returned and Marie knocked on the door about five minutes later.

"I'm so sorry, Marcy," she said apologetically as I opened the door.

"It happens," I said, trying to be gracious. "I was home to pick her up, so it all worked out all right."

"No, it doesn't happen. Not to me. I don't forget kids, I never have. I'll find a way to make it up to her."

"Oh, you'll be buying Girl Scout cookies," I said. "She's been waiting to hit you up for a sale all day."

"I will, I'll buy a bunch," she replied.

The remainder of the visit was uneventful. Marie bought a bucket load of cookies, and we discussed the finalization process. Everything appeared to be fine until Marie was saying her goodbyes and Hannah dropped a bombshell.

"Okay," Marie said. "The next time I see you may be in court to finalize."

"Yep, between the fifteenth and twenty-fifth," Hannah replied. Jon and I looked at her in stunned silence.

"That's what you told me," she said to Marie. "Between the fifteenth and twenty-fifth we'll finalize."

"Uhh…," Marie began to stammer, her eyes wide and mouth open. Surely, she didn't give specific time constraint. We have no control over this situation and no idea what roadblocks may come up in this final month. There was still distant birth family who had made sporadic contact with Hannah. Who knew if moments before we were supposed to sign the papers someone would object? And besides all that, anyone in their right mind knows to never give a child a specific time frame on something this important. There are always factors that can't be controlled.

"As long as the paperwork comes in by then," I interjected. "We don't have any control of the paperwork."

"That's right," said Marie. "I can do everything perfect, but it may take the state longer to do the paperwork."

Let the damage control begin. That was Friday. By Saturday we were feeling the effects of the uncertainty and concern that the visit had stirred up in Hannah. One of the most common reports from anyone who has adopted an older child is that they will have episodes of testing you to see if you're going to be true to your word and stick with them. After all, adults who claimed to love them in their past have proven that when times got tough, they weren't willing to put in the effort and love it takes to be a parent. When Hannah started to test, she got mean and the tantrums flew while Jon and I tried to hang on for dear life.

Saturday morning started out like any other. We had a late breakfast and decided to check out a local pond for ice skating in the afternoon. The pond ice was perfect and the three of us were enjoying the day together, playing hockey with pine cones and racing across the ice with our dogs. But as time wore on and unbeknownst to us, her frustration level began to rise. It started off with simple gloves. She had pulled them off to adjust her skate and asked for my help to put them back on. The whole winter we had battled with gloves, coats, and boots. She would ask for help, refuse to take it, become frustrated, lose her temper, and end up in a tantrum. So I tried to preface the situation with some boundaries before helping.

"Sure, I'll help you," I said. "But here's the deal. You put your first glove on, and I'll show you some tricks for the second. If you try it and still can't get them both on, I'll get it on for you." She glared at me. Deep breath in and steady yourself.

She got the first glove on and looked at me for assistance.

"Okay," I said. "Here's a trick that helps me when I'm playing in the snow." I demonstrated how to pull down the sleeve of my jacket and hold it while slipping on my glove so that my wrist is protected from the cold.

She glared at me and began jerking her sleeve and throwing her glove. "Okay, I'll give you a minute to take a break, and then I'll come back and help you if you need help," I said and skated away for a minute. I watched her take some deep breaths to calm herself, and when she appeared to have cooled down a bit, I skated back over to help her.

"Are you ready to give it a shot?" I asked.

"I can't do it," she replied.

"Yes, you can. I'll show you again, and if it's not working, I'll help you get your glove on." Again, she glared at me. I showed her how to put the glove on, then removed my own to assist her with getting hers on. She pulled her arm away.

"Mine doesn't work like that!" she yelled.

"What doesn't work?" I asked.

She sighed in anger and began pulling her sleeve and throwing her glove again.

"Would you like my help?" I asked, keeping my voice calm and level.

"It doesn't work like that! I can't do it!"

"You can too. Just show me what doesn't work."

She stifled a scream and began throwing her gloves.

"Hannah, you have a choice to make. You can take my help or we can go home. I'll give you a minute to think about it," I said and skated away. She continued to stay seated on the ice and was soon brimming to full-tantrum level.

I looked at Jon. "I think it's time to go home."

"Yeah, we've been here for a while, and I know I'm getting tired," he said.

"Me too," I replied.

"I don't want to go!" Hannah screamed.

"Well, we think it's time," said Jon, and I skated toward the shoreline to remove my skates. Jon stayed near her, coaxing her up, and by the time I had my skates off, she was standing. Then to my astonishment, she started stomping off the ice. It's hard enough to skate on pond ice, let alone stomp.

"Hannah," I said as she got to the shore. "You will not stomp your feet. Do you understand me? That is not allowed at home and is certainly not allowed here. Now knock it off."

She threw around her boots and skates, her cheeks red with anger.

"You go on ahead," Jon said to me. So I took the dogs and walked the trail out to the car and waited. And waited. About twenty minutes later, Jon arrived with a tear-streaked Hannah. As we drove toward home, the car was permeated with silence. We had been doing so well as far as the behaviors were concerned. No major tantrums to speak of, and then this one, which bordered on the brink of toppling all others.

"I'm sorry," I heard a small voice in the backseat say.

"What are you sorry for?" I asked.

"For yelling," Hannah replied.

"And what else?" I asked.

"For throwing stuff."

"And?"

"I don't know," she replied.

"Well, were you respectful to me?" I asked.

"No," she said.

"Were you respectful to yourself?"

"No."

"Did you let me help you?"

"No."

"I want you to think about those things for a while," I said as we finished the drive home. When we reached the house, Hannah grabbed her things and took the dogs inside while I helped Jon clean out the rest of the truck.

"What did you say to her?" he asked me.

"What?" I said, astonished that he was questioning what had happened.

"She said you wouldn't help her and that she feels like you don't care about her. What did you say?" I stood there dumbfounded.

"I asked her to try and put her glove on and if she couldn't get it, then I would help her. She refused to do that," I said icily. "I tried multiple times to help her, but she would not listen or let me."

"Okay, that's what I thought. You just need to talk to her."

Inside I went and sat at the kitchen table, asking Jon and Hannah to do the same.

"Hannah," I asked. "Did you ask me to help you?"

She nodded.

"Did I show you how to put your glove on?" Again, she nodded. "Did I ask you to try and put your glove, and that if you couldn't get it, I would help you get it on?" She looked away, her head confirming her response.

"See, the thing is, that's not what you told Abba, is it?" Her eyes widened and she looked at the table.

"Abba just told me that you told him I refused to help you. Is that true?" She shook her head to say no.

"Hannah, do I care about you?" She nodded yes.

"So how does it make me look when you tell Abba that I wouldn't help you?" I received a shoulder shrug in response.

"You know how it looks," Jon said. She refused to meet my eyes.

"It makes me look really bad, doesn't it?" I asked. "It makes me look mean, and like I don't care at all, doesn't it?" She nodded.

"So was that a lie?" Jon asked and she nodded yes and began to cry.

I took her into my arms. "I love you," I said, and she cried harder. After a few minutes, I drew her back to look at me.

"So we know that you lied. But another thing is that you didn't take responsibility for your actions. When you didn't get your way and had a tantrum, you tried to make it look like my fault. That's not okay."

"Okay," she said.

"So what do we do now, Hannah?" I asked and she shrugged her shoulders.

"Well, what do you think? We've tried lots of different things for lying and taking responsibility for our own actions, but it doesn't seem to be working."

"We want to help you, Hannah," Jon said. "So what will help you learn and remember next time something like this happens?"

"I don't know," she said.

"What about a code word?" asked Jon. "Like we know that when you're starting to get frustrated, we take a break and cool off. How about when someone isn't taking responsibility for their actions, we just stop and say something like "responsibility," then we all take a ten-second break where no one talks and think about it."

"That sounds good," Hannah replied.

"All right," Jon stated. "We'll start with that and see how it works." Hannah nodded in agreement.

Though we moved passed the main event, Hannah continued poor behavior throughout the day. She was sassy and rude and downright mean for most of the afternoon. Lucky for me, most of it was directed my way. By five, I was at my wit's end.

"Why don't you go have a girls' night with some of your friends?" Jon said. "Get away from the house and take some time for yourself." God bless him. I was on the phone with a girlfriend in less than thirty seconds. When Hannah learned I was leaving, she was disappointed. She had been wanting to have a family sleep-out and was hoping to do it that night.

"We're not going to stay up late and do the sleep out tonight, huh?" she asked as Jon and I were warming ourselves in front of the fire while I waited to meet my friends.

"No, not tonight," we replied.

"Because you're going to be gone," she said and she pointed at me.

"No, Hannah. That's not why," Jon said.

"Why do you think we're not going to do it tonight?" I asked.

"Because I was mea—didn't behave good today."

"You were right, you were mean today," I replied. This was new. No one had ever called her mean before, and she was the first to recognize her own actions. "Fun stuff like a sleep-out is earned. You had a rough day today, but that needs to change tomorrow, okay?"

"Okay," she said.

"We love you," Jon and I said. "And we want us all to be happy, so we need to remember to treat others how we want to be treated."

"I'll kiss you good night when I get home," I said as I pecked her cheek and headed toward the door and a slice of sanity.

The next day was better, but throughout the week, we continued to have episodes of tantrums, huge amounts of attitude. We were all struggling to get through each day and praying the next would be better.

I found that my new job became my solace as I became closer and closer friends with Jamie, one of my coworkers. Jamie has two daughters, just a couple years older than Hannah and had dealt with many of the same issues with her oldest that we were facing with Hannah. She became a great sounding board and confidant. It was wonderful to finally have a friend who seemed to understand some of what we were dealing with and offer helpful advice.

On that Thursday Jamie told me of an upcoming Broadway production of *Annie* that was coming to Spokane that weekend. I knew Hannah would absolutely love it. After all, she spends most of her waking moments singing, and her nightly fifteen minutes of reading is done opera style. When I was about her age, *Annie* was one of my favorite movies. I watched it all the time. Jane thought she would enjoy it and encouraged me to take her.

"I saw *Annie* when I was eight and absolutely loved it!" she said.

So that night I went home and broached the subject with Jon.

"Guess what's coming to Spokane?" I asked him.

"What?"

"*Annie!*"

"Oh," he said. "That would be fun for you two."

I laughed. "That's about what I figured you'd say. I think Hannah would love it, though."

"Oh, absolutely. You should take her," he replied.

"Yeah, I don't know. Her behavior hasn't exactly been great lately."

"I know, but I think the two of you need a chance to spend some quality time together," Jon said.

"Quite honestly, and I hate to say this, but I'm terrified to take her."

"Yeah?" Jon inquired.

"Yeah. She's been so mean to me in every way. I'm afraid to spend six hours alone with her in the car. What if she keeps acting like she has? And on top of that, I really don't feel like she's earned the privilege."

"But maybe that's why you should take her, so the two of you can have some fun away from home. Some bonding over a big event."

"You're probably right. And I know she would absolutely love it. I'm just nervous. And that makes me so frustrated! I shouldn't be afraid to take my daughter to a special event and I am."

"All the more reason to go."

So that night at dinner I brought it up to Hannah, wanting to feel out the idea before making any promises.

"Hannah," I asked, "have you ever seen the movie *Annie*."

"Uh, no," she replied.

"It's this really cool show about a girl named Annie who lives in an orphanage and meets really neat people, and there's lots of singing and dancing."

"Huh," she stated. So much for the interest I had hoped for.

"The musical is going to be in Billings this weekend," Jon said.

"I used to watch the movie of *Annie* when I was your age, and I really liked it," I said.

No response.

"Going to a show like that would be really special, and a really big deal," Jon said, trying to perk some enthusiasm. "I don't think she knows what to expect," he whispered to me.

"Imma was thinking maybe the two of you could go and have a girls' day on Saturday. You could go to the show and check out Spokane. It would be a really special day."

"Oh."

"Would you like to go see it?" I asked, brimming with the hope that she would show some excitement at the prospect. After all, this was something I would have never been able to do as a child, but would have died for the opportunity. But Hannah was not me. She had not had the same childhood I had, and so her understanding of what a big deal this would be was lost to her, and the excitement I so wanted was lost to me.

"Sure," she said hesitantly. I felt defeated. But I wasn't giving up yet. I knew she would love it in her own time.

After dinner I looked up *Annie* online and began watching some clips of the performance.

"Whatcha doin'?" Hannah asked, coming over to the computer.

"I'm looking at some of the *Annie* songs. Want to see?" I asked, pulling up "Hard Knock Life."

She climbed into my lap and appeared to finally be showing some interest in the play. Over the next couple of days, Jon played up how special a day this was going to be, and that it is a big privilege to be able to go. And I prayed it would be a good day.

By Friday night she was getting excited, and my nerves were calming some. We discussed what we would wear; after all, one has to dress up when going to the theatre, and she picked out a skirt and sweater with tights. Saturday morning she was climbing in my bed by seven asking, "Imma, what time do we leave for Spokane?"

By eight thirty we were on the road. It was an absolutely gorgeous day, hinting of spring but with the chilly bite of winter clinging to the air. The three-hour drive went blessedly well. She kept herself occupied with activities in the backseat, and we chatted as we drove down the highway to Hannah's first experience with Broadway.

We reached Billings early and decided to park in the downtown garage attached to one of the shopping centers, which also happened to be only a few blocks from the theatre.

"What is this?" she asked as I pulled onto the ramp entering the garage.

"This is a parking garage. See those windows there?" I asked, pointing to our left. "Those are stores in the mall. And on the lower level is a restaurant, that's where we'll go in and then head into the mall part of the building."

"Is this like a big circle?" she asked as we rounded the corners, looking for a parking space.

"Kind of. See the color stripe on the wall?" I nodded toward the blue stripe that turned yellow was we rounded a corner. "When we find a place to park, we'll have to remember which level we're on by what color the stripe is where we park." It was such a surreal experience to explain the mechanisms of a parking garage, something that I took for common knowledge but was such a new and fresh experience for Hannah. It was such a lovely feeling to realize the innocence and naivety of her youth.

Girl to the core, Hannah couldn't wait to hit the mall, especially since she realized there were escalators, or esqulators as she called them.

"Imma!" she cried in surprise laced with joy. "Can we go up the esqulator?"

"Yep. We're going to head into the mall and grab some lunch before we go to the show, so ride that one on up and then we'll find some place to eat."

So we road the escalator, and then it was time to find a restroom after our journey. Nordstrom's was the closest store with facilities and I wove Hannah through the designer jackets and dresses toward the back of the store.

"What's the lounge?" she asked, reading the sign on the lady's room door.

"That's the bathroom. It means it's pretty fancy."

"Wow," she said as we walked through the door. "Imma, there are couches in here!"

"Yep." I chuckled. "Pretty fancy, huh?"

We ate a quick lunch in the food court, stopped into some children's stores, and I had to drag her away from the shoes (truly a girl after my own heart), then we headed out the doors, after sampling the escalators a few more times, and started toward the theatre.

It was a beautiful day, the sun glistening down on us and warming our steps. We arrived at the theatre about half an hour before the show began, picked up our tickets from will-call, and talked the outdoor security guard into taking our picture in front of the *Annie* billboard. Then it was off to find our seats.

The building was packed, and we had to wait in an ocean of people before we made it to the ticket collector and could look for our seats. Hannah spent the first seven years of her life in a very small town, and our current home city was even smaller. Rarely had she been in a city as large as Spokane, and it was becoming apparent that all the excitement and people was beginning to unnerve her. I silently prayed that peace would calm her heart and hoped for the best.

Our tickets were for row R, seats 52 and 53. As we walked into the theatre, I pointed out the letter stamped into the side of each end seat of the rows and the number placed on the edge of each seat. I explained that each of the rows have a letter and go in order of the alphabet, starting with the first row.

"That's how we know where to sit," I explained. "We find the end seat marked with an 'R' and then walk down that row to seats 52 and 53."

We found our row, which happened to be the first one visible as we entered the theatre door, and then traveled down the row to our seats. Hannah was too excited and nervous to sit still, so she stood by her chair and examined the room. After a few minutes I noticed her tension mounting.

"Imma, we're in the wrong row," she said.

"Why do you think that?" I asked.

"I've counted three times, and this should be row P, not row R."

"Well, maybe the first couple rows were taken out for the orchestra," I said.

This did not suffice her, and she counted again, out loud.

"See," she said in exasperated worry, "this is row P, not row R."

"Okay, remember when we came in and we looked at the letter on the end of our row? It was marked 'R,' so we're all right. And if for some reason we're not, all we have to do is move back a couple rows."

She sat down in a huff of irritation. I let her be for a bit, hoping she would take the time to calm herself down. Soon short notes of music flitted to our ears as the members of the orchestra settled into their places and began tuning their instruments.

"What are they doing?" she asked in an irritated voice.

"That's the orchestra," I said. "See that light down at the front of the theatre? Below that light is called the orchestra pit. That's were the musicians play from."

"There's real people playing the music?" she asked in astonishment.

"Sure is. They'll do all the music for the whole play. And all the actresses and actors will sing themselves too."

"Wow," she said, and I hoped that maybe she was beginning to understand the significance of this production.

As the curtain dropped and the first notes of the music filled the air, she sat back in her seat and crossed her arms. Maybe she wasn't as impressed or excited as I had hoped, I thought.

It took some time, but finally the play drew her in, and soon she was captivated by the set and the performers.

"It looks like a movie!" she whispered as the scenes changed. By intermission she was hooked and the rest of the play held her rapt attention. By the time the curtain closed, she was astounded by the skill of the actors and all signs of frustration and anger had dissipated.

"Imma, that was awesome!" she exclaimed as the house lights came up. I breathed a sigh of relief. "So those were like professional actors?"

"They sure were," I replied.

"Even the kids? They get paid to do this?"

"Mmm," I said, smiling. "Want to go see the orchestra pit?"

"Yeah!"

So we made our way through the crowds fighting to get out of the theatre, to the front and peered over the edge of the pit. I pointed out the various instruments and sheet music while she stared.

"So if someone accidentally dropped something down there, then could they go into the pit?"

"You may not drop anything down there," I replied.

"Oh, darnit!" she said, and we made our way back to the doors and out into the late afternoon sun.

As we walked back toward the garage, she was alight with the excitement and energy of the play. She skipped and danced down the side walk and asked questions about the actors, story, and anything else she could think of. When we reached a crosswalk guarded by a blinking red hand, she spotted traffic meters along the side walk.

"Imma, what are those?" she asked, pointing to the pay meters.

"That's a parking meter," I said. "Have you never seen one of those before?"

"Nope."

"That means that people have to pay to park there," I explained.

"Wow, lots of people had to pay to park!" she exclaimed.

"Honey," I said with a smile, "so did we."

"Ooohh," she said, the knowledge of city life and things new and unknown breaking into her small-town girl mentality.

We rode the "esqulator" one more time before making it to the garage, following the yellow line to our car, and hitting the highway for home. After driving about half an hour, we decided to stop for dinner. We chatted and worked on the kid's menu activities while waiting for our meal.

"So," I asked, "do you want to be a Broadway actress now?" I was sure that this experience would have the thrill of the stage beckoning her toward stardom. The answer she gave shocked me. Her face blanched and her eyes grew huge as she shook her head.

"No way," she said. "Imma, that would be way too scary!"

"Really?" I laughed. Since when had my little social butterfly ever been afraid of drama?

"All those people? Uh-uh. But if I *had* to play someone, know who it would be?" she asked gleefully.

"Who?"

"Mrs. Hannagan! So I could be mean!" She giggled. Well, there you go. Not Annie or Ms. Grace, but Mrs. Hannagan, the villain. Lord help us.

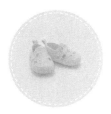

THE BIG DAY!

Those six months seemed to stretch forever, but finally all of the paperwork of our paper pregnancy had been signed, sent, and notarized, and we could finally finalize our adoption. Though I knew that plenty of people wanted to share in our incredible moment, my heart was still warmed and overjoyed as I walked into the conference room and so many faces greeted me. Jeff and Marie were waiting patiently with Sharron, Jason, and Rainey. It soon became apparent that though I had said we had a large party and the courthouse attempted to compromise, it was still a standing-room-only event. Within minutes Brenda, the clerk of court, walked in, followed by the judge.

"All right, I need Mom and Dad and Hannah up here in these three seats," Brenda said, pointing to the group of three chairs in front of a long table.

"All right, folks, I'm Judge McKade. You must be Jon and Marcy and Hannah," Judge McKade said as he sat down across the table from us. "Brenda's going to swear you in and then we can get started."

"You three stand up and raise your right hand," directed Brenda. We stood and listened as Brenda asked and solemnly sore to tell the truth and nothing but it.

"Yes," said Jon.

"I do," I replied. And Hannah nodded.

"Okay then," began Judge McKade. "In the matter of Hannah set before us today. Do you two understand that this will make Hannah your legal responsibility? You will be required to clothe and feed her and she will be eligible for inheritance?"

"We do," Jon and I answered.

"How does that sound to you, Hannah? They been good to you?" She nodded, her shy eyes cast down to the table.

"All right then. I hereby announce Hannah Jane Hanson," he said with a smile and stood up. "You guys want to take a picture?"

I'm a big fan of parties. I think they should happen at any occasion you can think of, and this was an occasion! So after the festivities, our family and friends all joined us back at our house to celebrate. After enjoying some great food and wonderful company, Hannah sought me out in the kitchen. "Now we don't have to worry anymore," she said, looking up at me. "Because you raised your hand and made a promise to the judge, so now no one can ever take me away."

She said two sentences, but a volume was spoken. All these months knowing how she had fretted and stressed over the permanence of our situation. Understanding how frightened she was that this too would not last, while at the same time praying that our reassurances would help. Now she could finally take a deep breath without the restriction of uncertainty wrapped tightly around her. Now we were truly a family forever.

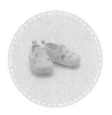

ALMOST BABY

While I knew that adopting would never quell my desire to have a baby, I had hoped it would lessen it. And for a while, it did. Things progressed slowly with Hannah as we transitioned from foster-adopt parents to a legally linked family. Jon and I became better at learning the triggers for tantrums and redirecting the acting out, but we were far from perfect. I took solace in the verse from Lamentations, the one where it says that God's love for us is new every day. It kind of became my mantra. Each day was a new day and each day I had to learn how to be a better mom, just as Hannah was learning what it was like to truly be a part of our family. Yet even though things were crazy and emotionally trying, I still wanted a baby.

While I knew that baby fever had never completely left, it wasn't until about a year after we had Hannah with us that it took hold again, full force. My sister Mindy and her family had moved to Pennsylvania and, as a result, had never met Hannah before. I was dying for her to meet her cousins and to spend some much-needed time with my big sis, so Jon and I saved for months and watched for deals on airfare. After a few weeks of monitoring every flight website I could find, the best deal came along and I booked our tickets back East. I was so excited I didn't know what to do with myself, and Hannah was just as thrilled to make the trip and meet more of her new family. It only sweetened the deal that Mindy's oldest daughter, Meagan, is in the same grade and the girls had spent time trying to get to know each other the old-fashioned way: good ole snail mail.

The morning of our flight, we crawled in the car before God woke up and drove the two hours to the airport to catch our flight. It was Hannah's first time in a jet, and she was thrilled to be making the trip. After finagling our luggage and shuffling seats with some of the other passengers a bit (who knew they don't seat you together when you purchase more than one ticket? Stupid airlines.), we settled in for the uneventful flight to Pennsylvania. My sister and Meagan were waiting for us at the terminal, and it was such a wonderful feeling to finally be able to hug my sister again! Then I got to do something I had wanted to do for years: introduce her to my daughter. Hannah and Meagan hit it off from the first minute they met and quickly scrambled into the backseat of the car for the ride to Mindy's house. I hadn't seen my sister's family in over two years, and it was a shock to me how much they had grown. Apparently we looked a little different too. My nephew Halden said as much.

"What do you mean?" I asked him.

"I don't know. You just look like a mom," he replied. What better compliment could there have been?

The rest of our trip was great. We did all the fun touristy things like go to the zoo and museums. And all the fun family things like watching soccer games and staying up late to chat. I hadn't been feeling very well, and Mindy asked if I thought I might be pregnant, but I assured her it was highly unlikely. The time went by way too fast, and before I knew it, it was time to go home. We said an incredibly tearful good-bye, and then we were off, back across the country to our home in Montana.

We were just starting to settle in the routine of being home when a few afternoons later, Jon called me from work. I could tell he was unsuccessfully trying to contain some serious excitement.

"What is going on?" I asked, laughing at his lack of restraint.

"Marie just called me, and I probably shouldn't be telling you this, actually she told me to wait to say anything, but I couldn't."

"What are you talking about?" I asked, my anticipation rising as well.

"She said there may be a baby that needs a home. Apparently a girl in Polson is in the hospital. She just had a baby boy and they don't think she's going to keep it, but hasn't done any adoption stuff, so they called DPHHS."

"Are you serious? What are we supposed to do? What can we do?" I was shocked into hopeful anticipation. We wanted a baby so bad, but had resigned ourselves to the fact that it wouldn't happen through foster care. There just didn't seem to be any way unless you took a child as only foster parents first, and I didn't have the heart or emotional ability to give a baby back. Could this actually be a chance to have an infant?

"Well, she said to wait for her call, and she'd let us know what was going on when she had more information." Right. Like I could wait around for the phone to ring. We all know how patient I am.

"I'll call her," I said.

"I knew you would," he replied with a smile in his voice.

She answered on the third wring. "Hi, Marie, it's Marcy." And she laughed.

"I knew he wouldn't be able to keep a secret. Okay, here's the deal. Now don't get excited." Sure, like that was possible. "There is a baby boy that was born this morning, but his mom wants to terminate rights. We're not sure where the dad is, but he seems to have been out of the picture for quite a while."

"Is he native?" I asked. Knowing that if the answer was yes, there was little-to-no possibility of this going our way. Any time there is a child with links to the tribe, the tribe has first say as to what happens with their placement and 9.9 out of 10, it's with a tribal family.

"No, he's not," she replied. "But there are a couple other families being considered for his placement, so I need to know where you guys stand."

"We're in." No hesitation.

"What about baby supplies?" she asked.

"Well, there's a Walmart in Polson. I'll pick up whatever we need there when we pick him up. And our families will pitch in anything else that comes up."

"What about your job?"

"If this works, I just became a stay-at-home mom."

"That's what I thought you would say." She laughed. "All right, well, I'll keep you up to date. Nothing is anywhere near official yet, but I wanted you guys to be prepared in case anything comes through. So now we wait."

I thanked her and hung up the phone. Then I dialed my mom and Mindy for some moral support. They started doing what I had been since I hung up with Jon: praying. And hard. About three hours later, I received a call back from Marie. By the tone of her voice, I could tell that it wasn't good news.

"I'm sorry," she said. "Because there was no reason for the child to be removed from the mother's care, DPHHS couldn't take custody of the baby."

"But she didn't want him," I said, dumfounded.

"I know, but it doesn't work that way. She had done nothing to endanger his life and was in fact trying to make the best decision for him, so the state says we can't get involved. The hospital is trying to link her with a private adoption agency."

Just like that, he was gone. Just like that, my heart was broken. Just like that, I was grieving again. It was like I had miscarried. In all reality, I had. This was an emotional miscarriage, just like I had faced so many times before. And it was a wake-up call that even though I had thought my heart had healed, it didn't take much to rip that wound back to gaping open.

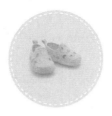

STARTING OVER

About this time Hannah started hinting that she wanted more siblings. She knew we were not able to adopt Rainey, though we would have loved to, and she was ready to have some more kids in the house and started dropping hints. Soon we went from "It would be fun to have another kid" to "I want another sister. Or a brother," and then that "we need two more kids, and then we can stop." and Jon and I were starting to feel like it was time to start looking into adding more kiddos to our family as well. While we were still foster licensed, we also hadn't given up the idea of having biological children as well. I had stopped taking the pill about a year before this, and with my constant irregularities and symptoms, I was right back to where I was before. To add to that hope, I had completely revamped my lifestyle. I started cutting out white flours and sugars, changing my diet to more whole grains and fruits and vegetables. Though I had always been active, I had also started integrating running into my routine and was building up on miles and speed slowly but surely. Yet I was still chubby, and nothing seemed to be changing that. My PCOS was also still out of control, so I decided to started looking into medicinal ways to manage it since obviously diet and exercise weren't doing it.

I made an appointment with a friend of mine and former coworker who prescribed Metformin to try and battle potential insulin resistance due to the PCOS. Within the first two weeks on the lowest dose of the medication, I lost six pounds, more than I had lost in the entire three months previous. I was so excited! Not only does Metformin work to control insulin levels, it's also an ovulation booster. The more I read about it and its use in PCOS, the more I found that many women were able to get knocked up with just this alone. Could it be I had found my miracle drug? I so hoped so!

But like all things, as soon as my body became tolerant of the Metformin, I stopped losing weight and didn't find continued success until maxing out on the dosage. While it did help control the insulin resistance, it didn't seem to be helping the cysts or plunge me into an ovulatory state. So my friend referred me to a specialist in Missoula. By this time I had lost thirty pounds and was feeling pretty healthy and proud of myself. I was eating right, exercising, and it shouldn't be hard to get pregnant now, I thought. So I went to this new appointment with high hopes.

Unfortunately, living in the sticks means you have to drive at least two hours to reach civilization or specialized medical care (or Costco, or Safeway, or a theatre, or a mall), but I had driven longer than that and was ready to tackle this infertility with a new fervor. I was grossly disappointed. Let's start from the beginning, and I'll fill you in.

After the two-hour drive, I waited in the waiting room forever. Not a new thing, but still irritating. Then I was ushered into a tiny room where the nurse/medical assistant took my vital signs and asked me all the initial personal questions. Then I waited for the doctor. Most patient rooms in a doc's office have soothing paint or wallpaper and a smattering of magazines. This one was wallpapered in pink flowers circa 1984 and the only magazines in sight had to do with horses and hunting dogs. I kid you not. Awesome. Then the doc came in, all five foot seven inches and ninety-five pounds of her, and she gave me the look. You know the look. The one a health care provider gives you as they size up their perception of your health and compare it with their own size 2. That look. I am not a size 2 and quite frankly never want to be. But it was apparent that she thought I should be and I knew this wasn't going to end well.

After the sizing up, on both sides at this point, she got down to the nitty-gritty as to why I was there and started asking more questions to take my history. When we got to how many children I had and I answered one, she scribbled down the number and made some comment regarding the fact that I could get pregnant at least once. When I told her my daughter was adopted, she scratched her number out. Huh. Now I was getting kind of cranky. Just because my child isn't biological doesn't make her any less my child. Put that number one back on your little patient note there, lady. But she didn't, and the questioning continued, and as it did, her tone became more and more high and mighty. Then she asked me about my eating and exercise habits, which I told her, and she responded (and I write this exactly how she said it), "Well, if you would just get your weight under control, you'd be fine." To which I responded by reminding her that I had lost thirty pounds and was quite fit. Really? Your answer is to call me fat? That's the cure all for this? Oh, I was hot. I'm pretty sure our appointment ended there and she could ride her horse right out of my life, with her hunting dogs at her heals.

So I found a new doctor, who I loved. My first visit she spent over an hour just talking with me, learning about my history and my story. Then she was ready to get things rolling, ensuring me that she had worked with many PCOS patients, and she had confidence that I could get pregnant. So I started all over again. This time I wasn't leaving it all to the doctors. We were still licensed, and I was still advocating for our family and other kids who were still in the system.

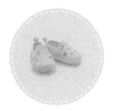

HISTORY HAS A WAY OF REPEATING ITSELF

Trying to get pregnant again, wholeheartedly, meant reliving all the emotions and pain that I had before. I thought that having a child would have made it easier, but in all actuality, it made things worse. We were at a time in our lives when it seemed like everyone around us was pregnant or just had a baby (well, whenever you're trying to get pregnant, that's what it feels like). What I realized was that though yes, we did have a child, we never had the opportunity to bond with her as new parents bond with an infant. We had missed so much of the vital aspects of her childhood and as a result were trying to catch up on the eight years of our absence. As insignificant as that may sound, it's a big deal. We had never had the option to bond with our child and build the fundamental foundations of trust, love, and respect. As a result, we were in a constant state of flux and insecurity within our relationships as parents and a family. Just because you place a child into your home doesn't mean that all the past hurts and losses are magically erased and life is a bountiful basket of goodness. Parenthood in a normal situation is work, and this type of parenting is far more complex and integrated. So as I was again popping Clomid and testing for ovulation, wishing I had been a fundamental part of Hannah's infancy and toddlerhood, my friends were kissing their new babies good night and posting ultrasound pictures on Facebook.

After four months of not thinking I had ovulated, I suddenly became extremely nauseated and, after two weeks, was facing the glimmer of hope that maybe this time the culmination of weight loss, exercise, and pharmaceutical intervention would finally result in that pretty pink + in the EPT window. But I started spotting a tiny bit, so I gave it a couple more days. When still no real action going on, I called my doc who told me to get a pregnancy test. Down to the pharmacy I went and picked up yet another pregnancy test (those little buggers are so expensive! I mean, it's pee for crying out loud). And guess what? Yep, negative. I called her back to see if she wanted me to take a med to get things rolling in the cramp department, but she thought I should get a blood draw pregnancy test first. I drove the thirty miles to the hospital (because it's after hours and I'd have to wait up to a week for the mail in results from the clinic) where the lab tech draws from my hand (ouch!), then head home to a call from my doc saying this test is negative as well. So let's count it up how many things/times I got my hopes up: (1) late period, (2) nausea times two weeks, (3) taking a home pregnancy test, (4) taking a serum pregnancy test. How many mind-blowingly painful negatives did I get? Four. And one giant, throbbing goose egg bruise on my hand from the blood draw. Guess what I did next? I climbed in bed and sobbed.

Then I got mad, because that's apparently what I do when I'm really upset. I was mad at the doctor for wanting me to get two different pregnancy tests when deep down I knew they would be negative and full of false hope. I was mad at my body for not cooperating just for once in my life. I was mad at God for the usual reasons. And I was mad at Jon, because doctor after doctor and year after year, he had refused to go and get tested for fertility himself. Granted I understood his hesitations. It's embarrassing for one, and he's a pretty personal person. And it's scary as hell for another. No matter how much neither of us has ever laid blame, you still don't want the lack of children in your lives to be "your fault." Still, I climbed up in the stirrups and been poked, prodded, bruised, and pumped with drugs for years, and he had never taken the one simple step to rule out so much of our potential problem. Each time I brought it up, he promised to get tested. Each time my doctor asked about it, I made up an excuse. Though we had an amazing relationship, this was one area that threatened to create a canyon between us that might never be repaired.

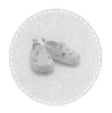

SO CLOSE BUT
SO FAR AWAY

As I continued to battle things emotionally and physically, we were still actively searching to expand our family through adoption. Things started to look good when Marie approached me about one of my former clients. When I had worked as a children's mental health case manager, I had a little boy on my case load who was about three and who instantly stole my heart. He looked so much like my nephew Eli that I couldn't help but find him adorable, and his family story was so horrendous that I instantly wanted to protect him. By this point, in January of 2010, my former client had aged a few years and worked his way in and out of the system. Initially Marie thought they were going to place him for adoption, and Jon and I stated our interest in taking him into our family immediately. But as so often happens within the system, things changed quickly and it was decided that he would be placed with a distant relative instead. Chalk up another emotional miscarriage, I was heartbroken.

Then my mother-in-law called, bubbling over with excitement. A friend of hers had confided in her that she was pregnant. This wasn't your standard pregnancy. She and her husband had been through some hard times and she had ended up having an affair. This baby was likely the product of that affair, and if so, she was seriously considering placing the child for adoption and attempting to reconcile things with her husband. Being a friend of Linda's, she had heard and was familiar with our story and had asked her if she thought we would be interested in adopting her child. Well, all right, now Linda wasn't the only one bubbling over with excitement too! Not only was there a baby coming, but a birth mom who was interested in us already! Now all we had to do was wait for a few months, a paternity test, and the final decision of Linda's friend. I was ecstatic and trying so hard not to get my hopes up. Jon was not so ecstatic.

"I told her not to tell you about it!" he said.

"Why?" I asked, puzzled beyond belief. Why would he want to keep something so potentially fabulous from me?

"Because. She hasn't made up her mind yet. She wants to get a paternity test and won't do that until the baby is born. What if it really is her husband's? She's not going to give it up for adoption then, and then we're out a baby. Again. I know how hard that is for you, and I didn't want you to get your hopes up. So I told her not to tell you."

Well, now I wished she hadn't told me too! After all, it was only January and the baby wasn't even due until May. Though I tried not to get my hopes up, I couldn't help it and would occasionally ask about the baby when talking to Linda to see if any decisions had been made. As the weeks wore on, it became more and more apparent that adoption was becoming an option of the past for Linda's friend. Soon we had a concrete answer: she would be keeping the baby. It's after things like this that I would wonder how much God thought I could handle. This was the countless child he had placed in my life and in my heart as a possibility, only to crush the hope. After so many disappointments, I wasn't sure if I could handle another false hope.

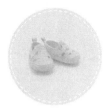

MYSTERIOUS WAYS

I've said before that if you want to make God laugh, you tell him your plans. I stand behind that 100 percent. I also think that he works in mysterious ways that I may never understand, and I don't believe in coincidences—it's all done for a reason. That's why the story of our second adoption is a little surreal. It all started about a year before we adopted Hannah. I was working my final year of nursing school as a student nurse/medical assistant at a small clinic and made some pretty good friends there. One of my coworkers, Wendy, had been a confidante through some of our struggle to conceive, and then again in trying to adopt, and she knew everyone in town (which isn't hard when town has about two thousand people). One day we were chatting in her office when an elderly lady pushing a stroller with two little ones in it walked by outside her window.

She turned right to me and said, "Marcy, you need to have those babies."

"What do you mean?" I asked, puzzled. They looked to me to be clean and healthy and with a grandma for sure. So what could be the problem?

"Well, that little boy and girl are twins, six months old, and are living with their grandma, who has to be in her seventies."

"What about their parents?" I asked. "Oh, I don't think it's a good situation, but I don't think they're in foster care either."

About that time we had a new patient come in and I left her office to do an intake assessment follow-up with our other clients. I didn't think much of our conversation, figuring that if CPS wasn't involved, and the kids were in the care of a stable adult, they probably wouldn't be. I finished out the day and went home to my hubby. I casually mentioned the twins to him that night over dinner, but we both knew there wasn't really much to be done. Wishful thinking hadn't gotten us pregnant or a child yet, and it probably wouldn't now.

The next night after work we made a trip to the grocery store to pick up the necessities and some Hot Tamales for a little cinnamon treat. Standing in line at the check-out I couldn't help but notice when a little red-headed grandma pulled up behind us, pushing a double stroller with two little ones in it. The little fair-skinned boy had bright blue-green eyes and blond hair while the little girl was olive complete with dark hair and deep brown eyes. They were lovely, and Grandma was all smiles when I said so. I asked how old they were and she said her little precious babies were six months.

Okay, now let me interject a little bit of the crazy that happens when you so desperately want babies. The things that go through your mind in a situation like this, or many others for that matter, are far from rational. Here's a few. *Huh, well if she's raising them, the parents must be out of the picture. I wonder if she'd give them to me. Can you imagine? Nope, I can't. She could like, just look at me and say, "You two look like a nice couple, want to have my grandkids?" Yeah, that would be pretty awesome. Reality check: not gonna happen. Yeah, well, a girl can hope.* And so on. Like I said, it's not so rational, but a girl can wish. Needless to say, she didn't offer me her grandchildren. Duh. She didn't know us from Adam. I turned around, paid for our goods, and as Jon and I walked to the parking lot, I told him that those were the twins Wendy had told us about. He commented something along the lines of "cute kids" and "she's taking care of them? Must have her hands full."

And we went home, pushing the thought of twins to the back of our minds.

The funny thing about twins is that they run in both our families. I have brothers who are twins, my aunt and uncle had twins, and Jon's aunt had twins. In my family, the joke was always wondering who among us kids would have them. Well, at this point, all of my siblings were done procreating, and no twins showed up. Since it didn't seem to be happening for us, the thought of another set of twins in the family seemed out of the picture. Until I went to work one day and my dear friend Karen had an idea.

Let me tell you a little about Karen. She's incredible. One of the strongest and funniest people I know and probably one of the biggest hearts as well. I swear she is on every committee that does good things in the county, from 4H to Relay for Life, and she knows more about WIC, maternal and baby health and immunizations than pretty much anyone I know. And she was one of the biggest advocates for us to find more babes to adopt.

I came to work one Monday and Karen started telling me that one of her church members Lynn has these grandbabies who are twins, and she needs to find a home for them.

"She's had the twins on and off since they were born. They lived with her for the first six months or so, and then she sent them off to live with another family, former foster parents, who have had them for the last year and a half or so. Well, this other family has four kids of their own and decided that they couldn't take care of the twins anymore, so they gave them back. But Lynn is seventy-three and those babies are babies and have a lot of energy, so she's looking for a home for them."

"Really?" I asked. "Like to adopt them?"

"I think so. So I told her she needs to give those babies to the Hansons," Karen said.

"You said what?" I asked, laughing and feeling my hopes start to glimmer and rise.

"I told her she needs to give them to you. And I gave her your phone number. What do you think?"

"Holy crap! Um, oh my gosh!" I said, dumfounded that this could maybe, possibly, really happen. "Yeah, oh thank you, Karen!"

"Well, yeah. Those kids need a good home, and you've got one," she replied. "So she's probably going to call you and you guys can work it out from there."

"Okay," I said, still a little shell shocked. Sure enough, later that afternoon I received a call from Lynn and we set up a time for her and the twins to come over and have lunch with Jon and me. I called Jon ecstatic, explaining the events of the afternoon.

"Are you serious?!" he asked, just as shocked as I was.

"Yeah, I am. And she's coming over for lunch on Thursday so we can have a chance to meet her and the twins and see how everything goes. I set it up for Saturday so Hannah wouldn't be there. I don't want her to know about anything just yet, because the last thing she needs in her life is another loss."

"No kidding," Jon replied. "I agree. Let's keep this on the down-low until we know a little more. So how old are they?"

"I think they just turned three. Sounded like their birthday was in the middle or end of May. Wouldn't it be crazy if it was the fourteenth like mine?" I asked.

"Yeah, it would. I don't even know what their names are!" He laughed.

"I know. It's all happening so fast!" I giggled. "His name's Logan and hers is Julia."

"Well, all right then. So what's the deal with rights and termination and all that jazz?"

"I have no idea," I said. "I'm guessing Grandma has full custody, but I know there was another family involved so I don't know what the details are with that. I guess we'll find out on Thursday."

Though it was only two days away, Thursday couldn't come fast enough for Jon and me. When Lynn pulled up in her white minivan, it was all I could do not to go hug those little ones close!

I made a simple lunch of grilled cheese sandwiches, and though they seemed small for their age, Logan and Julia had no problem finishing them off and then climbing in Jon and my laps to play.

"Well, they sure are settling in!" Lynn laughed, looking a bit relieved to see everything going so well. "I wanted to come today to see how they would take to you two, and they seem to be taking just fine!"

Jon and I both smiled. They sure did! But there was a long ways to go and a lot of questions to be answered before any of this could keep going.

"So what is the story on parental rights and what not?" I asked. "Where are their birth parents now?"

"Oh dear." Lynn sighed. "It's been a mess." Jon and I glanced at each other, sending a silent *that doesn't sound good.* "Doug, my son, and Tina are in Hawaii. They have been since the babies were about six months old. But they haven't seen them at all since then and I don't get regular phone calls either. I don't even know where on the islands they're at now."

"Do they still have parental rights though?" Jon asked.

"Well, yes, and so do I. I made sure they sign me up with third-party parental rights before they left," she replied. "That way I can do everything that they could do and take care of them just the same."

"So what about the family they lived with for a while? How did that work?" I asked. This was seemingly rather spider-webby and I was getting confused and concerned.

"Oh, the Markuses?" she asked. I knew that name. They had been foster parents and had taken care of some of the clients I had with the mental health center. "Well, I gave them guardianship so that they could take the twins to the doctor and everything if they needed too. But I still have and had custody just like their parents."

"So Doug, Tina, and you have parental rights. Do the Markuses still have guardianship?" I asked.

"Well, yes. They have to get rid of that where they are in Washington. See they moved right when I gave them the twins. Well, that day really."

"How did they end up with the twins? Were they placed through foster care?" I asked.

"Oh no," she said. "I gave them the babies. I knew him from before when Doug had had troubles. He's a cop you know. And he just fell in love with those babies." She smiled, recalling the memory. "Every time I saw him or he had to come out to the house, he just doted on them. So when I knew I wasn't going to be able to take care of them, I thought the Markuses would be a perfect family."

"So they were moving to Washington and took the twins with them when they left?" Jon asked.

"They sure did. She drove up with her car all packed up and I buckled them in and then off they went! It was so hard to watch them go, and they were so far away I could only go and visit once," she said.

"So they had them for a year and a half, why did they send them back?" I asked.

"Well, they had four children of their own. One was just a newborn when they took the twins, and I think it was just too much for them."

Jon and I exchanged a look. How could you take two babies, have them for a year and a half, and then just give them back? Neither of us could comprehend that. There's no way we would be able to do such a thing, which was the big reason why we wouldn't just be foster parents. The thought of having them as our own and then giving them back was just unbearable.

"Well, and Logan is really active," she said. "I think he has that ADD, but the doctor won't give him anything for it yet. So I have some vitamins that I give him, little dino things that are supposed to calm him down. But you know kids, you can't give one of them something and not the other!" She laughed. "So I give Logan one and then Julia gets one too. It really does seem to help."

Oh dear Lord, I thought. He's only just three! Of course he's active! I have some serious issues with ADD/ADHD meds to begin with. I know that for some kids it's necessary, but for most, the behavior is about something that is missing in their lives. And this seemed to be one of those cases. The twins, though appearing healthy, were definitely lagging in some developmental areas. They had not started potty training, though they were three. Neither knew any numbers or letters, barely any colors and definitely not shapes. She had a bit of a language issue, but that was likely do to age. And he was definitely active, though it looked more like nervous energy than anything.

"So what exactly are you looking for?" I asked. It seemed a little odd that there were so many routes of guardianship. I wasn't quite sure she had the same thing we had in mind.

"Well, I want a good Christian family to raise them," Lynn said.

"But do you want them to be adopted?" Jon asked.

"Well now, I don't know," Lynn replied. "I still want guardianship. I'm their grandma."

"Well, that's not something we're willing to do," I said, obviously taking her aback. "If we take these children, we will be their parents, and we will need full legal rights to them. That means that Doug and Tina's rights will be terminated and yours as well. Everything with the Marcukes needs to be cleaned up too. We have no problem with you still being in their lives as grandma, but we would be the parents."

"Oh," she said. "Well, what about Hannah's family? Do they still see her?" Lynn asked.

"Yeah, they do," Jon said. "She has a grandma and a little sister that she stays in contact with. She talks to them on the phone all the time, and we try and get them together at least once a month." That seemed to put her a little more at ease.

"Well, I guess that would work," Lynn said. "As long as I still get to be in their lives. I want the best for them, and they need a mom and dad. In a good home."

"All right, so now we need to figure out all of the legal stuff," I said. This opened a whole new pail of troubles. It seemed like everything was pretty complicated as far as guardianship and rights were concerned. But it turned out CPS had been involved at one point, and the regional director, who had also been involved in Hannah's case, had worked on theirs as well. After lunch, when it was apparent naptime was in order, Jon and I kissed and hugged the twins good-bye and Lynn drove off to take them home.

"Do you realize who they are?" I asked Jon as they were driving away.

"No, who?"

"They're the twins Wendy told me about all those years ago. The ones she said were meant to be ours. How crazy is that?"

"That's pretty nuts," he said, shaking his head.

Well, what do you think?" I asked.

"I think it's a long shot," he said. "There's a whole lot of legal crap and rights haven't even been terminated or started to be terminated."

"Yeah, I know. I'll call Shannon, the regional CPS director, and get the lowdown." And as soon as he went back to work, that's what I did. What I found out just irritated me, though I should have expected it.

The twins were born about five weeks early, and Julia's meconium (her first poop) tested positive for opiates. Turns out Tina, who had scattered at best prenatal care, also had a history of drug use. Her story was that she had a legit prescription for the opiates because she had been experiencing severe back pain. It was never really proven that this wasn't the case, as she had supposedly seen a doc in Idaho, but the circumstances seemed pretty sketchy and not so likely that this was the one and only time she had used during the pregnancy. It seemed even sketchier when the hospital had to put an order out not allowing Doug, Tina, or Lynn on the nursery floor because after CPS had placed them in temporary custody while ruling out the drug issues, the trio had tried to take them from the hospital. This little escapade intensified CPS's concerns and when they were ready to leave medical care, they were placed in foster care for about six weeks. Then CPS ruled that they could be returned to Doug and Tina because the new parents were living with Lynn and therefore were in a stable environment. Here they stayed for six months, until Doug and Tina were ordered to court for drug charges, which they weren't too excited for. Instead of appearing in court, they jumped bail and ditched the mainland, heading for sunny Hawaii. We were informed we could see them on an episode of *Bounty Hunter* if we wanted, high, upstanding citizens as they are.

Before they flew the coop, they made Lynn a third-party parent, so no further action was made in their case and it had been closed. The twins were in a stable and loving environment, and the state was happy. When I asked Shannon what steps we should take next, she recommended that Lynn call her and we could start working through some of the legal mess. She warned me, it was likely going to be messy and take some time. Rights hadn't been terminated and to do so, the state would have to try and contact the parents. This may bring them back into the picture. As ominous as this all sounded and appeared, and it did appear pretty ominous, I had a good feeling about Logan and Julia. Those babies were meant to be mine. Even Wendy had said so all those years ago.

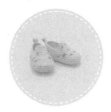

LET THE GAMES BEGIN

After that first lunch date, we started taking the twins on the weekends, giving Lynn a break and us a chance to see how this might work. We told Hannah about them after our first meeting and kept it pretty light: we were going to be helping out with some little ones. They might be staying with us for a bit, and we'd just take it from there. She knew some of the complexities of dealing with rights and termination and all that, but we also assured her that if we took kids into our home on a long-term basis, it would be for adoption. She didn't need another loss in her life, and quite frankly, neither did we.

Our first weekend with them was Memorial Day of 2010. It was the start to a beautiful Montana summer, and to kick things off, we decided to go camping with Jon's cousin Nick and his family. He and his wife, Hanni, and their kids, Avery and Zephy, are some of our dearest friends, and we were excited to share this new possibility with them. So we packed up our things, loaded the boats and coolers, and took Hannah and the twins for our first family campout. We had a great time. The kids played and swam, roasted marshmallows, and went for walks. It was a great opportunity for us to learn more about Logan and Julia.

One thing we noticed right off the bat was that Logan called any woman of childbearing age "mom". He called me mom, and he called Hanni mom too. That was going to be something to work on. The next thing we learned was that Logan had night terrors. That first night sleeping in the tent, Jon and I woke to him rocking in his sleeping bag, crying, and throwing his head into his pillow. I put my hand on his back, rubbing it in small gentle circles, murmuring calming words, and after a bit, he calmed down enough to lie back down. He was obviously asleep the whole time, but Jon and I still were heartbroken over the obvious fear that plagued him when he slept, especially when they night terrors reappeared each night as he slept.

At the end of the weekend, we returned Logan and Julia to Lynn. Handing them back was one of the hardest things I ever had to do. I told Jon that it felt like my children were missing. Law or no, rights or termination be damned, those were my babies and they needed to be in my home. The next weekend we took them again, only this time when we sent them home, they didn't do so well. Lynn called me about an hour after we dropped them off.

"Julia has been crying nonstop since you left," she said. "I don't know what to do. I can't get her to calm down."

"Do you want me to come out there?" I asked, my heart clenching at the thought of them being away.

"Oh, could you please?" And so I went, calmed her down, and kissed them good-bye again. Just as I had when we left Hannah those first few weeks, I left a bit of my heart behind. Meanwhile, the legal mumbo jumbo wasn't moving very far or very quickly. Lynn, Jon, Shannon, and I had all decided that the best way to go about this whole thing was through the foster system. Doing to the complexities of the multiple guardianships, the legal costs to try and get everything done, and getting them done correctly would likely be a fortune. On the other hand, if CPS took over, they could be placed with us as foster children, and the state could take care of all the legal processes as it needed to be done. This would also insure important needs like insurance were met. Before all this could happen, we had to have meeting after meeting.

Our first family group decision-making meeting occurred the end of June. This meeting comprised of Jon and I, Shannon, Lynn, a Mennonite family that often watched after the twins, and on the phone was Lynn's other son. Doug and Tina had been notified to call in as well. Tina told the caseworker who tracked her down that she would phone in, but never did. Doug, however, did make the call, though obviously intoxicated. He had some fantastic plans though. He was currently homeless, but was going to be moving into a house with some guys he was starting a band with. He was sure he could use his room as one for Logan and Julia as well.

Now hold on a minute. In order for me to take a child into my home, I had to meet pretty stringent requirements. I needed smoke alarms in every room, a room each for boys and girls, carbon monoxide detectors, regulations playing outside, fire drill maps, and the list goes on and on. I relayed this to Shannon, asking if he had to meet requirements as well.

"Well, yes," she said. "But nothing to the extent that you do."

"So I have to have all of these things, background checks and finger prints, but he could move them into a house with a bunch of random band members?" I replied.

"Technically, yes," she said, looking no more pleased than I was. I have no idea how she does it. Shannon is a smart, wonderful woman who sees the flaws in the system, but because that's how the system works, her hands are tied. It would drive me batty. I'd lose my ever-loving mind. Fortunatly Shannon, Jon, and I weren't the only ones to see that this was a monumentally crappy decision. Lynn's other son did as well and he took our defensive with Doug.

"Listen," he said. "You trusted these kids with Mom, and she's done a really good job. But she can't take care of them anymore. She's found a family that can, and she likes them and trusts them. You need to let them go. If you want to be a good dad, start by making that decision. Get out of their lives and let this family take over."

"I know," Doug said. Shocking us all. "You're right. If Mom trusts them, they must be good people." Holy crap! Could this actually be turning our way? The whole room seemed as shocked as we were.

"All right then, Doug," Shannon said. "I'll have papers sent to general delivery on the island. You just need to go in and sign them, put them back in the stamped and addressed envelope, and send them back. Are you willing to do that?"

"Yeah, I will. You just send them there and I'll take care of it," he said.

Jon and I looked at each other, shock resonating from our bodies. One down, one to go? Certainly it wouldn't be that easy. And it wasn't. Doug never showed up at general delivery, and he never signed the papers though they were sent multiple times. Tina never did either. She refused to talk with the worker when she called, insisting instead that her new boyfriend handle the calls, and she never picked up any paperwork to either contest or acquiesce. But the state moved forward. Lynn went to court and dismissed her rights, placing Logan and Julia in legal custody of the state, and on August 15, she drove them to their new home with Jon, Hannah, and me. We knew we still had a long road to travel, but at least Logan and Julia were where they were meant to be, with us.

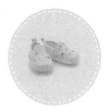

DELAYED? I THINK NOT

One of the things about adopting from foster care is that you have monthly (at least) visits from your social worker. They are there to monitor the children's progress and behaviors, see how they are adjusting and settling in, and just check on them and you in general. I hate it. Fortunately I've had great social workers. Marie and Shannon are wonderful women, and both truly care for the welfare of the kids they work with. Initially with the twins, we worked with Shannon only since she took the lead on the case, and Marie's primary focus was on adoption. That first visit with Shannon she read them books and we played with Play-Doh while she assessed where they were developmentally and asked Jon and me questions.

"I think we need to keep in mind that Julia tested positive for opiates at birth," Shannon said at her first visit. "I think they are behind a bit developmentally, and it may come into bigger play in the future."

"I don't know," I replied. "I think maybe they just haven't been worked with."

"I think they're bright," she said. "But it's something to keep in mind. Those little synapses could have been damaged in utero, and we don't know when or where that damage may show up."

Jon and I had a feeling about them though. And our feeling was that the Marcuses had obviously not worked with them at all. These were bright kids, that much we had seen in the short increments of time we had spent with them. It wasn't long before they were proving us right. By Shannon's next visit, three weeks from then, the twins were fully potty trained, could count to 10, know 95 percent of their letters, all of their colors, and most of their shapes. Shannon was astonished.

"So you think they just hadn't been worked with?" she asked me, a twinkle in her eye.

"I think they just hadn't been worked with," I replied.

While they were obviously incredibly smart, they definitely had some behavior issues too. We had expected as much. Not only were they just out of the terrible twos and into the monstrous threes, but they had had multiple disruptions as well. Logan's behavior really concerned us, as he would through huge temper tantrums, screaming and yelling at the top of his lungs. Then when he was really upset, he would take it out on Julia, pushing her or hitting her. By the end of each day, I was exhausted and at my wit's end. I tried everything from time-outs to time-ins to taking away certain toys, but the behavior continued. He showed other symptoms of attachment disorder as well. He had no stranger danger and would go to anyone, at any time. Especially if they were a grandmother type. This wasn't a huge surprise. In an effort to give herself some much-needed rest, Lynn evoked a long list of sitters. The twins would stay with various families, sometimes for days at a time. No wonder every adult woman was either "mom" or "grandma." It got to the point where I was terrified to take them in public. I never knew what would set off a huge tantrum or if he would stay right with me out in public.

Julia, on the other hand, was the exact opposite. It was pretty apparent that her goal was to stay under the radar as much as possible. Where he craved attention, she wanted nothing to do with it. She would sit on your lap if you picked her up and put her there, but she never climbed up on her own volition. Where he was dramatic and outright aggressive, she was passive aggressive. The girl could glare down with the best of them, and we wondered how long it would be before she really bonded with us, if ever.

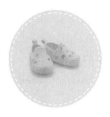

HAVE PATIENCE

It turned out it wouldn't be long at all before Julia truly bonded, but it certainly didn't happen how we had hoped or anticipated. No, not in the least. It all started on Hannah's birthday. The twins had been living with us for just under a month when Hannah turned ten. As is the case with most little girls, she wanted to have a sleep-over and Jon and I were happy to oblige. Since her birthday was on a Friday, it worked out perfectly, and before we knew it, we had a house full of tweens. The girls were giggling and laughing, playing their new band instruments, and getting ready to dive into the best part of sleepovers: gossip.

Jon decided the best thing he could do was get out of the house. What man in his right mind wants to be trapped with eight preteens, right? He loaded up the twins for a trip to the park and a drive in the woods. They hadn't been gone long and I was surprised when I heard him pulling up in front of the house, laying on the horn. But I didn't think much of it. The twins love it when he honks the horn, and it was getting chilly outside. They had probably just come home for warmer coats. But when Jon came running into the house, Julia in his arms, her hand wrapped in his sweatshirt and his face drained of color and full of panic, I knew something was wrong.

"She cut her finger," he said in that calm voice that comes in panic. "What do we need to do?"

My husband, bless him, doesn't do well with blood. The man can hunt and process with the best of them, but when it comes to people—he and blood don't mix. I, on the other hand, am a nurse, and not really phased by it, so I wasn't too concerned when he said she'd cut her finger. I thought surely it was something small; they had only gone to the park after all. So I pulled his sweatshirt off her hand and was shocked when I didn't just see a little cut. I saw the bone of her right index finger, where it had been completely severed from the tip of her finger at her first knuckle. Oh. Dear. God. I put the sweatshirt back over the hand of my child who wasn't even crying, looked at Jon, and said, "We're going to the hospital."

"Go back to the truck," I said, "and I'll get the girls to go to the neighbor across the street."

When I opened Hannah's door and told the girls that the party was going to have to move so we could take Julia to the hospital, they didn't believe me. Not until I pulled out the mom voice and told them to get moving. Then their eyes got wide and they made quick work of getting out the door. Poor Hannah. I felt so bad about her party! Fortunately our neighbor was also the mom of one of Hannah's guests and a good friend of mine. She swooped in and took over the party process, making sure that the girls had a great night.

Jon and I were not having such a great night. With Logan in the backseat and Julia on my lap, we drove the agonizing thirty miles to our local hospital. The whole time Jon was white-knuckled, trying to get us there safely and quickly, while Julia and I sang her favorite songs and tried to stay calm. She did amazing. She didn't even cry the whole way to the hospital.

When we arrived at the ER, they quickly got us in and rolling toward surgery. It was such a blessing that I had worked there previously and as such knew the entire surgical staff. As they whirled around taking x-rays and calling specialists, Julia and I sat on the bed, her on my lap, as I sang to her songs from *Bullfrogs and Butterflies*. What was even more of a blessing was when our surgical staff started singing too. They knew the songs from their childhood, as did I, and sang them to their own kids at home. During the whole ordeal, Julia only cried twice. The first time was when they removed her bandage to take an x-ray and she was able to see her finger. The second was when they gave her a shot to knock her out. That one ticked her off pretty good. But before long the drugs kicked in and she was singing too, as loud as her little voice would go, all the way back to the OR.

She pulled through surgery beautifully, and Jon and I were able to take her home that night. She slept in our room so that we could keep an eye on her, wary of the anesthesia, and she woke up bandaged and happy the next day. As I was getting her dressed, struggling to find a shirt that would allow for her bandaged hand to travel through the armhole, she looked at me with her big brown eyes and said, "Mom, do I have an owie?"

"Yeah, baby. You do," I said, trying not to cry.

"Aw." She grinned. "That's a bummer!"

Here she was, bandaged and broken, but smiling and happy. If this little girl wasn't a fighter, I didn't know who was. Looking back on it, this was really what changed our relationship with Julia. Where she had been determined and aloof before, she now had to be dependent on us, because she was hurt and learning how to compensate.

A few weeks later, I was brushing her hair and she looked at me out of the blue and said, "You're Mom, but you're not Mommy."

"Well," I said, trying to gauge how to work this one. I was sure that Mrs. Marcus had been Mommy, not only to Julia, but to all of the kids because they had always known her as such. Here Julia was trying to make the distinction between the two of us. She wanted me to be Mommy, but she wasn't sure if she if it was okay to do that or not. So I replied the only way I knew how.

"You can call me mommy if you want to," I said.

She gave me the biggest, most self-assured grin. "Okay," she said.

Later that week, Logan and I were in the kitchen when Julia walked in with a pair of ladybug rain boots.

"The other mommy gave me these," she said, holding the boots.

Logan cued right in. "Yeah, the other mommy, but she was a different mommy than you."

"Yes, your foster mom gave you those. I didn't. But you get to stay with Daddy and me forever now. You don't have to go to another mommy and daddy ever again."

Julia smiled. That was enough for her and all she needed to know. Logan is a bit more logical though, and this just got him thinking.

"We don't?" he asked.

"Nope, you don't. Daddy and I get to be your mommy and daddy forever, because you're going to be adopted."

"How do we get 'dopted?" he asked. Now he was really intrigued.

"Well, we go and see a judge and the judge asks if we want to be your parents forever and if you want to be our kids forever. We all say yes, and then you don't have to ever have another mommy and daddy. You get to stay with us until you're all grown up. Does that sound good?" I asked.

He gave me a big gap-toothed grinned and nodded. "We don't ever have to have another mommy and daddy?"

"Nope," I said.

"Cause we're gonna be 'dopted."

"Yep," I said. "Hannah is adopted too. She came to live with us and then we went to see a judge and she got to be adopted too so she gets to stay with us forever too."

This made him smile even more. "So Julia and me gonna be 'dopted just like Hannah!"

"You sure are," I said. And he gave me a great big hug then ran off to play. But Logan is a thinker. He likes to ask the same question as many different ways as he can, and he likes to process things over and over until they are just right. I swear that boy is going to be an engineer. Or a rocket scientist. Needless to say, this wouldn't be the end of our 'doption discussion. He would randomly ask again what it was and when it was going to happen, just trying to make sure that the answer was always the same.

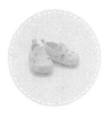

ULTIMATUMS

By October, things with the twins hadn't moved anywhere. Nothing had been filed as far as petitions to terminate rights, Doug and Tina were out in no man's land and out of contact. The twins were in our home, but nothing had been done to ensure their permanency. To top it off, I could count nine of my friends or family who were pregnant. I felt like my whole world was at a standstill and wasn't sure if things with the twins were ever going to lead to adoption. I was emotionally and physically exhausted and still popping Clomid and Metformin and peeing on ovulation testers. Jon still hadn't been tested. It had been eight years of trying to get pregnant, and he had never made that first move to rule out things on his end of the deal. I was sad, frustrated, and deeply, deeply hurt. Finally one night I lost it.

I had recently been in to see my doctor to get a new prescription for Clomid. She was sure she could get me pregnant and was still trying to rule all things out. Contrary to the former specialist, she was proud of my weight loss and dedication to running and other forms of aerobics. Best of all, she listened, and she wanted to know why Jon had never been tested. Each visit I had with her I made up another excuse and this time I was finally done.

"I don't know," I said when she asked me once again. "I know he's afraid, but I honestly don't know why he won't just do it." She gave me the supplies again for a sample and encouraged me to take him get things done. By this point, I was with her over the next couple of weeks I would ask him when he was going to get tested. Each time he gave me the same response, that he'd do it the next time he went to town. Every time he went, he neglected to follow through.

"I don't think you understand," I said one night as we were wrapping up the dishes after dinner. He had just gotten back from a trip to Kalispell and had again skipped the doctor's office. "I don't think you get what it does to me when you say you're going to get tested and then you don't."

"I'm sorry. I'll do it," he said.

"No," I said. "That's not enough. You don't get it. You don't get what it does to me."

"Yes, I do. I know you're upset," he replied.

"Then you just don't care?" I asked, tears filling my eyes.

"Baby, I care, I just. I don't know. It makes me uncomfortable."

"Oh, well then. I'm so sorry. I have no idea what that's like, being uncomfortable," I said, sarcasm lacing my tears with fury. "I can't tell you how many times I've been poked and prodded. All you have to do is jack off in a cup."

"Marcy," he started, reaching for me.

"No," I said, pulling away. "You just told me that you know how it makes me feel, but you do it anyway. So you obviously don't give a damn about my feelings."

"That's not true. I do care, a lot, more than you can imagine." This time it was his eyes getting misty as he spoke.

"Then I need you to know one thing. If you don't want to get tested, fine. Don't get tested. But you need to know that if you don't, I will never be OK."

"What do you mean?" he asked.

"I mean that there will always be this break between us, this canyon that will only get bigger as time goes on. I'll forgive you, eventually, but I'll never be able to forget that you weren't willing to do this for me, for us. Over time, I don't know what that will look like. I do know that I will never be fully OK with us. There will always be a break in our relationship."

"Okay," he said, his voice ragged with emotion. "Okay, I'll get tested." And he did. The results were inconclusive. Mostly normal, though he had an abnormal amount of round cells. My doc wasn't sure what the deal was with that, so she referred us to a urologist and Jon made an appointment. It didn't go well. The doctor was wretched, made Jon uncomfortable, and redid the exam twice while Jon was there. Jon said he felt like the guy didn't know what he was doing. He ordered some further tests for Jon to complete. Since we didn't much care for the urologist, Jon was going to complete the other tests and take all the results to a different doctor. He never did.

Meanwhile, things with the twins were still in limbo. We were working pretty closely with the former county attorney, who I loved. Unfortunately it was November and she was about to retire. At this point they were leaning toward filing for termination based on abandonment. They hadn't been able to do so before since Doug and Tina had left the twins with Lynn and given her a role in guardianship. Since she had terminated those rights and they were wards of the state now, Doug and Tina had six months to step in and try to make some steps toward reunification. If they didn't, the state could file on abandonment. She was hoping that could happen in December.

December came and went, and nothing seemed to be happening. It wasn't until February that things finally got pushed through paperwork-wise. The irony in that was that based on Montana law, if everything has been done and taken care of, we could have finalized their adoption in February. At this point we were just finally getting things going. Instead of rolling along smoothly (working with the government, remember?), we kept hitting roadblock after roadblock. The CA office submitted notices for Doug and Tina, and then they came back and said they didn't do it right. So they submitted new ones. Then they weren't published right. It happened again and again. Each time was supposed to start a three-week time period where Doug and Tina could contest. When we got yet another call saying things were being pushed back, Jon and I had had enough.

"We're going to go talk to them," I told Marie.

"What, like have a 'come to Jesus meeting' with the county attorney?" She laughed.

"Yep, pretty much," I said. I wasn't kidding. We were done. This may be their job, but the one thing that workers and court persons seem to forget was that this is our life and the lives of our children. Do your job and do it right. If I messed up as much as they had been, I would have lost my job by now and it was time someone be held accountable.

Our meeting lasted all of five minutes. The CA apologized and guaranteed that things would be done appropriately and correctly from now on. Jon and I were doubtful, but three weeks later, it seemed that all was well. The publication to appeal had run its course and no one seemed to be coming forward. We may just be able to move on with things after all, which was good, not only for the legalities, but because Jon had been offered a job in Washington and we couldn't legally move the kids out of Montana if they were still in foster care. We needed this thing wrapped up and ready to roll.

We started packing and trying to decide the best way to move forward as a family. We didn't want to be separated, and I certainly didn't want to be a single mom, so we decided that we would split things up a bit. Jon and Hannah would move to Washington so he could start work and she could round out the school year there, making some friends for the summer. Meanwhile the twins and I would stay residents of Montana and would travel back and forth between the states. Yeah, that looks great on paper. Until you read the paper that has your credit card bill on it, which has been wracked up with gas for the fifteen-hour trip each way. But we didn't have much of a choice. The twins had to stay Montana residents, as did Jon or I, and we still had monthly visits with the social worker. Now we were just biding time, waiting for everything to come through from the state.

We should have known that these final steps would follow in the footsteps of the rest of the journey: long and difficult. Though the CA had published the notices, when their three weeks of publication was finished, more paperwork had to be filed. This final document was to be submitted to the courts and was the last chance for Doug and Tina to file for appeal. Once this document was in place, they had thirty days to make their move. Well, as shocking as it seems, that paperwork wasn't filed. So while we were waiting and waiting and waiting, it didn't matter in the least. All of the legal steps hadn't been taken.

We found this out on May 11. That meant that though all previous legalities had been completed in February, we now had to wait until the second week of June before we could even file our adoption paperwork, and Doug and Tina still had their thirty days to appeal. This stress intensified when I talked to Lynn who said she had called Tina's mom and Tina was no longer in Hawaii, but back in Idaho and had asked about the twins. No one had heard from her in months, and now she was back in the area? Well, crap.

To top things off, our adoption paperwork hadn't shown up from the state and we were worried it had been lost. Fortunately it hadn't, but it had been sent to us and then back to Helena. Since we were moving and I handle the bills, I wanted all of our mail in one spot so I wouldn't miss anything. To do so I had everything forwarded to our new home in Washington. Turns out that documents from the state don't forward. When our adoption packet showed up at our mailbox and we were no longer there, it went back to Helena. So here we were, waiting for our paperwork, set back another thirty days, and Tina was back on the mainland.

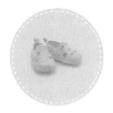

WONDER OF WONDER,
MIRACLE OF MIRACLES

At this point, we were definitely down to crunch time. To add to the stress, I constantly had this fear that Tina was suddenly going to take an interest in her biological children and try to appeal the termination. These fears came to a head just as our thirty-day wait was wrapping up. Three days before everything closed legally, Tina called Marie. Though she was out of the office, Tina left a vague message and a phone number, and Marie was legally obligated to call her back.

Jon and I were sick with fear. Surely, we hadn't made it this far only to have them ripped from us? But we knew that was entirely possible. We had friends who had been foster parents to children for longer than we had had the twins, assured that adoptions would go through, and crushed when the children were placed back with their parents. It could happen, it did happen, and we prayed beyond measure that it didn't happen to us. These were our children, they were meant to be from the start, and there was no way they were going back. I would fight this like none other if it came down to it.

Marie called her back. Tina didn't answer. Marie left a message. Then she called Tina's lawyer, left a message there as well. To our shock, awe, and prayerful praise, Tina never called back. Her thirty-day window was up, and we could finally file our paper-work and request a court date.

Here's the funny thing with court dates in small town Montana. Court only happens in our county on Tuesday. No really. Two different judges alternate Tuesdays to come to town and preside over hearings and legal matters. What that means is that when you file adoption paperwork, you also file for a Tuesday court date. Unfortunately, you don't pick which Tuesday you get, and you don't get to pick your judge. The computer that files your paperwork does. So here's what that meant to us: In order to file our paperwork, Jon and I both had to sign in front of a notary at our courthouse in Montana.

This meant that he would have to take time off work so that we could both be there (remember, this is June and he started work in April. Not a whole lot of time built up yet), and he would have to take further time off for the actual court date, whenever that would be. So we decided there was really only one thing we could do. We would drive home on Saturday, June 18, and pick up our packet on Monday, sign, notarize, and file for court. We would pray that the computer would pick the judge for the next day, Tuesday the twenty-first, so that we could finalize eve-rything, pack up the rest of our house, and officially move to Washington as a family. If it didn't work out this way, we would have to drive back to Washington, make another trip to Montana (which meant more time off work), and then pack up and hit the road for Washington again. (Remember how sad my credit card was with all the gas? Yeah, ouch.) So here we were, sitting with the odds stacked against us again. We did the only thing we could: we started praying. And so did our family, our friends, and anyone we happened to meet between that decision and the moment we filed our papers.

Marie was out of the office on Monday, but she left our adop-tion packet for us, and Jon and I quickly went to work figuring out everything we needed to do, where we were going to have to sign, and all the documentation we needed. When it was all in order, we made our way to the courthouse. Remember, this is a tiny town and I had worked in the courthouse before we moved, so everyone knew our story. When we handed the court clerk our paperwork and said we were hoping for a court date the next day, she was nervous with us and relayed her doubts that this would happen.

"I can't pick the date," she said. "It's all up to the computer. So let's see what we can do."

Jon and I held our breath as she tapped away at computer keys.

"Okay," she said. "Let's enter this part in." *Tap, tap.* "And now we hit this, and your judge is…" Her eyebrows rose and she smiled. "Judge McClain. She's here tomorrow and she has an opening at nine forty-five. I can't believe it."

Jon and I were both tearing up. "You have no idea how many people were praying," I said. "We'll see you at nine forty-five."

We were elated! I called my whole family, crying and laughing and telling them all to come on down, tomorrow we'll be finalizing it all and having a party! Unfortunately, I didn't have a thing in my house. Literally. We had either packed or moved everything but a card table and two camp chairs. Fortunately my dad had retired a couple months prior and my mom had made a massive amount of food, freezing what hadn't been used and had a bunch of leftover supplies as well. She packed up food and paper plates, plastic silver wear and cups and they headed to the party. Friends and family brought food, tables, and chairs, and before we knew it, we had a full house.

Our house wasn't the only thing that was full on Tuesday June 21, 2011. The courthouse room we had was packed as well. When the judge came in and all quieted down, she went through the usual questions, ensuring we knew what we were getting into, that we were willing to be responsible, and all that good stuff. Then she asked the twins what their names were and Logan said his full new name without a hitch. We had been talking to Logan and Julia about adoption and what it meant for quite a bit, and he understood it about as well as his little four-year-old mind could. But what he knew for certain was that it meant he never would have another mommy or daddy; he had a forever family. Before we knew it, the whole thing was over. As soon as those final papers were signed, it was like a huge weight was lifted off our shoulders, for all five of us. We could finally breathe and relax a little bit because now we were officially all Hansons.

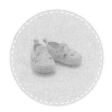

UNWRITTEN STORIES

It's funny to me that despite everything I've written, I keep getting comments from people to count my blessings and remember how blessed I am. But here's the deal: this outlet isn't about my blessings. It's not about the children I have through adoption. It's not about reaching beyond and becoming a better person thanks to the trials and tribulations of my life. It's not about constantly finding the positive, because quite frankly, that positive doesn't always exist. How can I say this, you ask? How can I systematically turn my back on my faith and beliefs and discredit the family that I have? Well, if those are the thoughts that come to your mind, you are precisely the person this chapter is written for. Because that's not what I've done. And if you truly read what I'm writing, or you've lived what I've described, you will recognize that.

Tell me, who do you know that's gone through infertility? How do you know their story? Is it because they struggled for so long and then were blessed by the miracle of conception? Is it because when all hope to conceive seemed lost and they decided to adopt, suddenly she becomes pregnant? It's a miracle, isn't it? Absolutely it is. I'll be the first to say so. But here's my point: you know their story because you've seen evidence of their success: a pregnancy and child. But do you know how many of us are out there that will never get pregnant? You will never hear our success story, because it will never be written. There are far too many of us to count. So like I said, I'm not looking for sympathy—I'm looking for understanding.

I'm pretty proud of myself at the moment. The week I had my surgery (which for those of you who know me closely know was *not* been a pleasant week), two of my friends had babies and I've found out that two more are pregnant. What does that have to do with me, you ask? Well, I'll tell you—I didn't cry. Not one tear was shed, when typically one of these notices would send me over the edge into a dark and desperate place. I was even told in person for one and I credit myself greatly for not breaking down right there in public. You may not realize this, but that's a *big deal*. Just ask my husband. Or any woman or couple who has fought infertility. I know women in their sixties who still break down at the news of a new pregnancy. Because the truth is, some wounds just don't heal. Or just when you think they have, that maybe, just maybe you can get through that baby shower or trip to the mall, something happens and your heart is re-broken.

But you have children! you say. How do you not see this gift that God gave you? you ask. Well, like I've said, this isn't about the blessings that I have. This is a whole different ballgame. Because contrary to popular belief, adopting a child doesn't ever take away the pain. It isn't a Band-Aid—nor should it be—to cover your grief. Why would you ever want one child to act as a replacement for another? That's just wrong. Adoption doesn't work that way.

A few chapters ago I asked you not to trivialize my pain. Please don't try to give me a Band-Aid for a gaping wound. Instead, try and learn my story so that you can be a friend for someone else. Instead, recognize that your friend who may be trying to heal may be an older woman and not your typical family starter. Remember that pain can't be classified, and if someone breaks down because you tell them you're pregnant, there is likely a whole other story to be told.

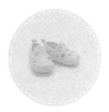

NEW DECISIONS

By August, after the adoption, I had an appointment with a new doctor in Washington. I transferred all my records and was hoping to maybe get some different answers with some new perspective. Now that things with Logan and Julia were finalized and we still didn't seem to be getting pregnant, I wasn't sure what I wanted to do. I knew that the medication, particularly the Clomid, wasn't good for me, especially with as long as I'd been taking it. It seemed that I had only two options: either continue being drugged up on meds that only made my cycts worse and gave me hot flashes or go for the gusto and have a hysterectomy. I had broached the topic of the latter with my doctor in Montana couple times, but she always redirected, saying that I was too young or to give this new cycle another try.

But I was getting emotionally and physically exhausted. Heck, I wasn't getting there; I'd been there for a long time. I didn't think I was going to be able to make it much longer. I went into my office visit with renewed hope and a refreshed mind, and I was pleasantly surprised. Dr. Fletcher was amazing. She really listened to my story and became familiar with my history. Finally she asked the big question.

"Are you wanting to get pregnant, Marcy?"

"Well," I said, "I don't know. I mean if it happened, I'd be ecstatic. But I really don't think it's going to happen anymore.

It's been a really long time, and I'm not sure I can handle all the emotions and the letdown anymore."

"I don't think you should have to," she said. "There is no reason you should have to be dealing with what you've been dealing with. All of the pain and all of the stress. Let's get you taken care of and better."

I was so relieved. I felt like I could finally say that I was tired, that I needed to stop, and someone would listen. We talked about a few different options, and she gave me some surgeries and alternatives to look into, including a new type of hysterectomy that uses a robot and results in a completely laparoscopic procedure. She told me that if I opted for a hysterectomy, this would be the best for me and gave me the contact information of a surgeon trained in this type of operation. Then she told me not to stress, to take my time, think things through, and call her with any questions.

"And if you want to go for it, we can always look toward next summer," she said. "That way it won't interfere as much with your work."

I really liked her. I gathered all the pamphlets and printouts and headed home.

"You've got until July to knock me up," I told Jon that night.

"Why, you think you really want to go through with surgery?" he asked. We had talked about the possibility of it before on a few occasions, but each time I had shied away, not really being ready to make that ultimate call.

"I don't know," I said honestly. "But I'm giving myself a year to decide. I really just don't think we're going to get pregnant."

"I know," he said, pulling me close. "I really don't think we are either."

"I mean, it's been almost ten years. If it was going to happen, I think it would have happened by now."

"Yeah, I think so too."

"So that's it. You've got almost a year to put a bun in this oven."

"All right," he said, laughing. And we left it at that.

Over the next few months I would bring up the topic on occasion. Each time we would talk through the pros and cons, with the pro side weighing heavier and heavier with each conversation. He always gave me the same response: he just wanted me to be happy, and he would support any decision I wanted to make.

As the months passed I went through some of the lowest times in this journey that I had ever had. We were shown the possibility of having a baby placed with us through foster care if we became licensed in Washington, but the classes didn't line up right with our schedules and it didn't work. I was so in, again, from the beginning. I even created a baby wish-list on Amazon, in case we did get all licensed and have a baby placed with us. Maybe we would finally get that baby shower after all. Then it seemed that we were in another round of baby mania. Everyone we knew was either pregnant or had a new little one. I felt like I was right back to where I had started. And it wasn't a good place.

As time progressed and I continued on the medication, I became stronger and stronger in my resolve to go for the full she-bang. In May I made called the doctor Dr. Fletching had referred me too, ensured that she was a preferred provider for my insurance, and made an appointment for an evaluation. Before I knew it Jon and I were making the two-and-a-half-hour drive to her office. (He keeps moving me to the sticks. I thought Washington would be better, but no deal.) Again we went over the pros and cons: no more emotional downers, no more meds, no more pain, no more of all the horrendous things that had been haunting us for the decade.

When I met the surgeon, Dr. Silver, I instantly liked her. She was calm and concise, and it was obvious that she wanted me to make this choice only if we thought it was the absolute best option for us. The more she learned our story, the more she agreed that it was.

"You've had a rough go of things, haven't you?" she asked after Jon had left the room and she was preparing for my exam.

"Yeah," I said. "We have. It's been really hard. And I just don't think I can do it any longer."

"All right, then. Let's get you taken care of and out of pain."

We scheduled my surgery for July 25, 2012. I had one more month before the baby maker officially closed up shop. I didn't hold out a whole lot of hope for that last miracle. And it's a good thing I didn't hold my breath.

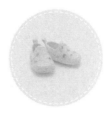

THE MOMMY CLUB

I did remarkably well (I think) when it came down to actually getting ready to go through with the operation. I had mentally and emotionally prepared myself as much as I possibly could and had finally decided that I was ready. It wasn't until about three nights before the surgery that I had a breakdown. It wasn't over what I had anticipated. I had known one would come before all was said and done, but I had always thought it would have to do with the finality of the surgery, that final step that said no way, no how, I would never get pregnant. That wasn't it. It was when I was Googling support systems and blogs for women who have had hysterectomies that I finally lost control.

Remember being in middle school and all the cool kids were in their own private club? They had the funny inside jokes and the coolest clothes and always seemed to be on everyone else's "it" list. Well, when you can't get pregnant, you feel like you're on the outside of the ultimate cool kid club. All the real moms can get pregnant. They get the baby showers and decorate the nursery. They have their own language of binkies and da-das, and they gather together to discuss the difficulties of labor and mid-night feedings. When you don't have that and are sitting on the sidelines, it's just like being back in middle school, begging for acceptance. Sometimes it's worse when you have adopted. Then every now and then a mom who doesn't know you're not part of the club will ask you about your personal experiences with pregnancy/labor/delivery/midnight feedings, etc., and then you have to tell them that you wouldn't know anything about that because you've never actually been pregnant or had an infant. Then it's their turn to respond. Let me tell you, it's not pretty. Most women haven't mastered the grace of taking information that completely surprises them and respond appropriately. Nope, not at all. Let me show you how it typically plays out:

Mommy 1: Oh, my pregnancy with little Emma was horrible! I had morning sickness the whole time and then my delivery was thirty-six hours. But I can't imagine you, having twins after all! I bet labor was just awful!

Me: Oh, actually I wouldn't know about the twins' delivery. My kids are all adopted.

Mommy 1(looking taken aback and typically actually taking a step back while her eyes become as wide as saucers and her nose get that tiny crinkle): Oh. Well, oh.

And at this point the conversation is typically over and she scrambles back to the inside mommy group and tries to forget. That's just one example. There are thousands more. I actually had one person who knows my story compare a situation to labor and ask for my confirmation in understanding. I just smiled and said, "I wouldn't know. I've never been in labor." That's why I'm writing this. Because no matter how many times we're in these conversations, the aftermath always results because people don't know what to say or how to respond.

So back to the mommy club. There have been multiple studies that focus on the desire to be a mother and really the fundamental part of our identity that it gives us as women. I'm kind of a science nerd, but I promise, I won't do nerdy on you. But it's true. Socially, there are major impacts on a woman's life and her family based on their culture and the general assumption that women become mothers. That's what we are supposed to do. So when we can't, it really is more than just a mental and emotional distress, it is a threat to our identity both personally and culturally as well. We all want to belong. We all want to be wanted and accepted. As a woman, we want to be part of the mommy club. When that's not possible, it reaches a part of us deep within our soul where our identity, our hopes, and our dreams are rooted.

Just like in middle school, when you can't make it with the cool kids, you go and join the ones most like you. For me, it was trying to build a community with others struggling with infertility. But there was so little out there! Blogs were as yet unheard of, and really the research was, and still is, pretty limited. But this is where I fit, so this is where I began to attach my identity. I wasn't in the mommy club, I was in the wanna-be club of the infertile. This is where I lived for nearly eleven years.

As my surgery date approached, I started to realize that maybe this wasn't going to be my club anymore. I could no longer say that we've been trying for X amount of years, because we wouldn't be trying anymore. I couldn't participate in the other blogs and forums for infertility where we discussed cycle changes and medications and sprinkled "baby dust" on each other through the working lines of the World Wide Web. I couldn't count my days and post about my uncertainty of whether or not this was a good time to buy a pregnancy test and maybe we had finally hit the jackpot. I was losing a physical part of myself, but I was saying good-bye to a huge part of my identity as well.

So as ridiculous as it sounds, I wasn't having a meltdown over saying good-bye to pregnancy. I was having a meltdown because I felt like I was losing such a major part of my identity. It was like getting kicked out of a really crappy club that you didn't want to be in in the first place, but it was the only one you sort of fit into to being thrown into another club where all the members are likely quite a bit older than you and very few understand the depth of what you've been through. That's not to minimize anyone else's pain or struggles, but the reality is, most women who have had a hysterectomy have also had children. Like I said, some of us never make it to the infertility success stories everyone seems so fond of, and sometimes, no matter how hard you try, you just can't make it into the cool club.

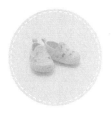

LOGIC DOESN'T
GUIDE THE HEART

It was about two weeks after my surgery when I had my first really difficult day. It was the first time since waking up from the anesthesia that I really cried for what I've lost. See, hubby and I were a little different from some when we tackled this whole infertility issue. I know my strengths and weaknesses, and I know my limits. For me I knew that I could never do procedures such as in vitro. There are multiple reasons that I couldn't. For one, the success rate of these procedures hovers right around 10 percent. Add a few zeros to that number and you've got a baseline cost, for one attempt. Second, I have some theological issues with it (just for me personally—I don't have any problem with other people choosing this route; it's just not within my comfort level). Here's why: I don't believe the body is meant to carry more than one or two (or possibly three) babies at one time. I'm not a Jon-and-Marcy-plus-eight type of girl. It's not good for your body to carry that many or to undergo all of the hormonal treatment necessary for cultivation and implantation. Also, I think that if God wanted me to have a bun in the oven, he'd set the dough out to rise. Third is my own mental and emotional state. I'm pretty tough, at least on the outside, but in this arena, things are a little different. Okay, a lot different. I recognized from the very start my frailty in regard to pregnancy and conception and I knew that 10 percent odds just aren't high enough to ensure my mental stability. One failed attempt and I would have been a goner. Now you might be thinking I'm being a little dramatic, but I'm not. I've said it before: I've been in some dark places throughout this journey, and I knew that with a failed attempt at something that invasive, I may not come out of that shadow.

Some people have looked down on me for that, for not trying everything. There have been times when I didn't feel like a good-enough woman because I wasn't willing to go those extra steps to try and become pregnant. It's like I had to defend my infertility. After all, we should have been doing everything possible, right? Sure, that's easy to say if you're loaded and/or never had a problem getting knocked up. I couldn't go that far. I knew that, and my hubby knows that, and neither of us was willing to make that compromise.

The same went for anything involving surrogacy as well. It really wasn't anything we had ever discussed because deep down we knew that it was never a route we would take. I'm not really sure why. I don't have anything against it at all, and for some it's a really viable option. It just never was for us. Maybe because we're both pretty territorial (I'm kind of a freakish momma bear—don't mess with my kids or my family. Any of them. Ever.) and just couldn't imagine having a part of us in someone else. I think for me it would come down to jealousy. I wouldn't be able to handle my child thinking someone else was her mother because of the voice she listened to her first nine months. Or not being able to feel my baby kick or get the hiccups because she was in someone else's womb. Or probably I'm just a territorial, jealous control freak. Yep, that's probably it. So surrogacy was never a topic of conversation. But…

Even though I know it would never happen, that we would never go for surrogacy, the thought was always in the back of my head that even though I was having a hysterectomy and partial oophorectomy, I would still have one ovary. So if it really came down to it, we could still have a biological child. I'm a pretty logical girl. I knew that we would never do go there, but still it was a calming center in the back of my mind. Then when I came out of surgery and Jon told me they had to take both ovaries, I wasn't upset. I gauged myself for emotion and it registered that I was okay with that. I knew that my doc was really conservative, and if she thought it needed to go, then it was completely necessary. Apparently (and a little surprisingly) I was all right with that. Until recovery day 12.

I hadn't had a breakdown since the surgery. I'd been really great with the realization that this was it, now it's done. I really haven't had any emotional ups and downs at all, which is pretty darn impressive since I was slammed into menopause (apparently my body hasn't noticed, and I'm not telling!). This day was different. I was talking with a friend of mine who just found out she was pregnant and we started discussing someone she knows who has been struggling with having a baby. She is so sweet and openhearted and it is so apparent that her heart is breaking for her friend, and in all that she isn't sure what to say or how to comfort her. I cannot tell you how much this warmed my heart. She is one of only a handful of friends who have come to me and said they know someone suffering from infertility and they just want to help, but don't know how. What a blessing these girls are to their family and friends! But I digress. Her friend had talked about surrogacy and my friend (bless her, she doesn't know my whole story or really anything about my surgery) asked if that was an option for us. Logically, I know it doesn't matter—surrogacy was never something we had really considered—but logic doesn't guide the heart. For the first time, verbally, I acknowledged that no, there was no further hope for us to have a baby. After I hung up the phone, I lost it. Logic or no, the pain was still there, and regardless of all the years and all the options, logic still didn't matter.

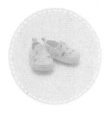

STILL A WOMAN

It's funny the things we work through in life. I've said before that we each have our own baggage, crosses to bear, and battles to fight. I am reminded of this more as I scroll through Facebook, looking at friends old and new and finding myself doing what I so often do, comparing myself to them. I think this is the curse of such social media outlets. While on one hand they are such a wonderful way to keep in touch with family and friends, they are also an excellent way to make yourself see all of the real and imaginary shortcomings of your own life. It's funny how even when you look at someone who you know has been through the wringer and back, I can still feel jealous. Why? Because they are swathed in that beautiful glow of motherhood and have a beautiful baby in their arms. No matter what horrendous things they've lived through, they have also accomplished that one goal that I never will regardless of what I have or haven't done.

Sometimes it almost comes as a shock to me that I'll never have babies. It's like I'm just walking along in my life, minding my own business when suddenly, one morning in the shower, I'm sucker punched by the knowledge that I will never carry a child. It's so shocking that at times it takes my breath away. I think the decision to have a hysterectomy and salpingo-oophorectomy is one that obviously doesn't come lightly, but it does have such drastically different meanings from one woman to the next.

I remember watching an episode of *Tool Time* with (cue the announcer voice) Tim the Toolman Taylor(!) where his wife had to have a hysterectomy. Before her surgery, she begged her physicians to leave her ovaries, but due to the nature of her condition, they were unable to do so. I was struck by her reaction to this. Her character was not only distraught at the knowledge that she was now completely and officially barren, but also that she felt like less of a woman.

Really, less of a woman? I hadn't thought of this before (granted when this show aired I was a preteen, but still). Why would losing this part of you make you feel like less of a woman? I never really got that, just like I've never understood why some men won't buck up and get a vasectomy when it's time to make birth control permanent. After all, it's a heck of a lot easier for them than it is for us. But regardless, this was a thought that fleetingly crossed my mind when I was preparing for my surgery. Would I feel like less of a woman when it was all said and done? I didn't think so, but still it was something that tickled at the back of my mind.

Fortunately, even after realizing that both my ovaries were gone and I had lost all my major reproductive organs, I still felt pretty womanly. After all, I couldn't see them to begin with, so outwardly I didn't appear any different. But I'm also the kind of girl who wears my battle scars like trophies. I have often wondered if I would feel the same if I was to have cancer and be forced to have a mastectomy. I don't think I'd feel like less of a woman. I think I'd be damn proud I made it. I can also say that having never been in that position, I could be totally wrong. Regardless, after my surgery I still felt like me—just a little lighter.

It wasn't until a few weeks after my surgery that the thought crossed my mind that Jon might see me differently now. We were at a party, chatting around a bonfire when I happened into Jon and a friend of ours' conversation. They were talking about parenthood and the possibility of more little ones when our friend brought up the topic of vasectomy. He was worried that having a vasectomy and no longer being able to have children would make him seem like less of a man to his wife. Huh. Hadn't thought of that. I looked to Jon and asked him if he thought I was less of a woman now. His response was pretty much what I had figured: a resounding "of course not" with a little bit of shock that I would even think such a thing. So I didn't feel like less of a woman, my husband didn't think I'm less of a woman, but still, isn't having babies what we, as women, are meant to do?

Here come those bourdons again. How do you carry something that in so many ways leaves you feeling exactly the same, but totally and completely different? I think each woman who makes this choice fights her own demons when it comes down to it, and I'm awed by how similar we may feel when deciding to end our ability to have children for once and for all. I think in each case there is a grieving and mourning for what might have been, regardless of whether or not you've given birth. For me it is such a bittersweet thing. For one, it is such a relief to finally release that hope that I've been holding for so long. Each month, regardless of where we were in our thoughts on getting knocked up, I still felt a quivering of hope. This became such an emotionally wearing state of being, to have and lose such hope on a regular basis that saying good-bye to ever having to wonder again was a relief. But I was also saying good-bye to such an integral part of who I am: a woman who desperately wants a baby. And I guess I haven't been completely successful at that, and likely never will be. No matter what I have in my life, I will always grieve for the pregnancy that never came to be. When it's all said and done, I think the only things I can really be happy to leave behind are the pain, the frustration, and the tampon isle.

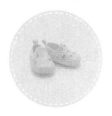

DREAM A
LITTLE DREAM

Dreaming seems to be such a mystical thing. There are songs about dreams, poetry pondering the dreams of the heart and mind, books about understanding them, and the list goes on. They say that dreaming is your mind's way of compartmentalizing things, putting all the pieces and puzzles of the day in order while the rest of your body drifts into dreamland. It makes sense then that over our years of trying to conceive, I've dreamed about babies more than you can imagine.

Of the countless number of dreams I've had over my life, the ones about babies have impressed themselves on my mind more than any of the other. One that has lasted with me for years is really just a snippet. I remember dreaming it was Christmas time, and we were shopping at the mall. I had gone to one end of the building to shop for presents and was heading back towards JC Penny and the Buckle when I caught sight of my hubby. But it wasn't just him. On his shoulders was a little one about eighteen months old. I knew she was a girl, though her fine blond hair was really just a bit of peach fuzz on her head, and she was wearing a little footy outfit. It was white, with a button at the top covering the scratchy zipper and small pink flowers scattered on the fabric. Her bright blue eyes were smiling as she rode on her daddy's shoulders, gripping his fingers in her little hands. That's all I remember, just that small scrap of what I thought would one day be. There have been so many others. My mind's imagination has run wild with scenarios of life after delivery.

It wasn't until the last few years that I stopped dreaming about having babies and started dreaming about adopting them. It was typically the same story line. We would happen into a situation where there was an infant and it would miraculously work out that that child would come home with us as our own. Last night I had this dream. I don't remember the exact scenario and much of what I remember is vague, but I do know it was someone we knew fairly well who had a baby, but wasn't going to keep him. I remember the feeling that came over me when this little boy's birth mom placed him in my arms, wrapped in a white blanket with a blue line around the edge. I told someone in the room that he was mine and I felt such a sense of overpowering emotions as I looked at his scrunchy little old-man-newborn face. It's a little ironic that I had this dream last night, considering today I went to a post-op appointment for my surgery. I suppose it's pretty understandable that my dreams of giving birth have ended and focus now solely on adoption. After all, my children are all adopted and that's really the only way we will ever have more children. I'm sure the knowledge of this impending appointment stimulated my brain into compartmentalizing as it does. Sometimes it still hits me that I'll never be pregnant. Ever. Not once.

Today was another one of those days, with the sight of this little one in my memory and the long trip to the doctor's (someday I will live again in civilization where I don't have to drive nearly three hours for a checkup. Just sayin'.). It's funny, though, how at peace with the whole thing I've been. I've only had a few moments of meltdowns where I've been sucker punched by the realization, and I don't think that's too bad. I'm pretty proud of me. I didn't even shed a tear when the nurse asked me today how many pregnancies I'd had before the surgery (Um, that would be none, a big fat zero on that score board). I shared this with my doc today, who followed up with her perspective on how she doesn't know how we deal with it, meaning the whole infertility struggle. She relayed her experience as a resident, knowing the women who would come in so hopeful again and again, only to be let down. Every time they come into the office they are surrounded by women who are pregnant or have new babies, and how horrible she felt knowing how heartbroken these women must be. And she's right, it is heartbreaking. I think that's why I'm so at peace now. (Well, today at least. Ask me tomorrow and you may get a different story.) I've allowed myself to let go, to give up that hope that was continuously raised and then broken down again. I've given myself the chance to love what I have, without continuously trying for something that ultimately was never going to be.

Sometimes I feel like infertility won. The big, bad monstrous beast that wielded its wretched head landed the final blow that knocked me down for the count. I guess in some ways it did. I will never be pregnant. I will never see my little girl with blue eyes and wispy blond hair gripping my husband's fingers while riding on his shoulders. I will be a lifelong member of the infertility club (membership is pretty pricey and comes with multiple hormonal imbalances, but hey, at least we all understand each other). But I'm still here, and I'm still fighting, and today that's all I can do, and that's all that matters.

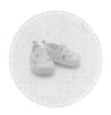

TAKE CARE

Well, that's my story, the good the bad and the ugly of it. I'm so glad you made this little trip with me. I hope that it was helpful to you. If you've never dealt with infertility, I hope that you now understand it a little better and can be the support system that someone else needs. I hope that this gives the husbands out there a better understanding of what their wives are going through—the secret battles that they face every month that go far beyond PMS. I hope this gives all the friends out there the courage to be a shoulder to cry on and an understanding heart to recognize the pain and joy we feel when you announce your upcoming pregnancy.

Most of all, if you're in the infertility club, I hope that this has given you a little hope and encouragement that you're not alone. You're feelings aren't insignificant because the insurance company doesn't think you have a problem or your friends and family don't understand how to be there for you. Your pain is real and substantial, and though you feel desperately alone, please remember that you are not. You are welcome in this place, and I hope that you can find that peace and solace your heart so desperately craves. If you would like to join in a community of your fellow sisters, you are welcome to log on to the No Maybe Baby blog (http://nomaybebaby.blogspot.com). Feel free to read the posts and join in with your own stories through the comment sections or the guestbook. If you would like a more confidential approach, you are welcome to message or e-mail me through the site as well. I would be happy to talk, vent, or cry with you.

I hope to hear from you soon.

Take care.